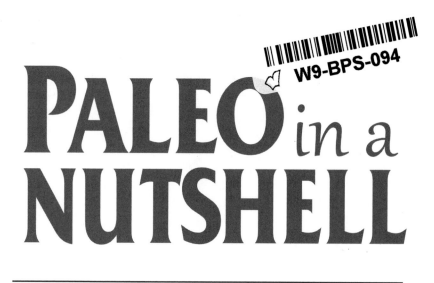

PALEO in a
NUTSHELL

Living and Eating the
Way Nature Intended

GEOFF BOND

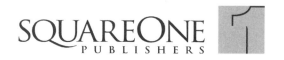

SQUAREONE
PUBLISHERS

The information and advice contained in this book are based upon the research and the personal and professional experiences of the author. They are not intended as a substitute for consulting with a health care professional. The publisher and author are not responsible for any adverse effects or consequences resulting from the use of any of the suggestions, preparations, or procedures discussed in this book. All matters pertaining to your physical health should be supervised by a health care professional. It is a sign of wisdom, not cowardice, to seek a second or third opinion.

COVER DESIGNER: Jeannie Tudor
EDITOR: Caroline Smith
TYPESETTER: Gary A. Rosenberg

Square One Publishers
115 Herricks Road
Garden City Park, NY 11040
(516) 535-2010 • (877) 900-BOOK
www.squareonepublishers.com

Library of Congress Cataloging-in-Publication Data
Names: Bond, Geoff, author.
Title: Paleo in a nutshell : living & eating the way nature intended / by Geoff Bond.
Description: Garden City Park, NY : Square One Publishers, [2017] | Includes bibliographical references and index. | At head of title: A simple guide to understanding and practicing the paleo diet and lifestyle."
Identifiers: LCCN 2017001269 (print) | LCCN 2017005264 (ebook) | ISBN 9780757004506 (pbk. : alk. paper) | ISBN 9780757054501
Subjects: LCSH: Diet. | Nutrition. | Prehistoric peoples—Nutrition. | Self-care, Health.
Classification: LCC RM222.2 .B6156 2017 (print) | LCC RM222.2 (ebook) | DDC 613.2—dc23
LC record available at https://lccn.loc.gov/2017001269

Printed in the United States of America

10   9   8   7   6   5   4   3   2   1

Contents

To my children—
who carry the torch down the generations.
"I see you stand like greyhounds in the slips,
Straining upon the start. The game's afoot:
Follow your spirit . . .!"

Acknowledgments

This book is the culmination of a long journey. Many people have helped me along the way and it is my pleasure here to single out some of them for special mention.

An early, and essential, influence was that of my quietly determined, selfless grandmother, Anna. At her knee, we learned to respect our bodies and to keep close to nature. She taught us to think critically about what we put in our mouths and to get plenty of fresh air, exercise, and sunshine. She pluckily challenged the dietary doctrines of her day. She was decades ahead of her time and, as pioneers do, had to suffer much uncomprehending banter. Thanks to her influence in my childhood over half a century ago, I have lived a life brimming with good health. If I have seen further than most, then it is only because, as a small boy, I used to sit on Anna's shoulders. She would be immensely proud.

My insights would not have been possible without the peculiarities of upbringing that created in me an untamed questioning, a delight in discovery, and a distaste for humbug. Thank you, then, to my undoctrinaire parents who taught me to be honest to the evidence and to hold fast in the teeth of dogma-driven opposition.

I am indebted to my wife Nicole. This book had a long and difficult gestation and she was always there with her encouragement and support. Like the faery's child, she found me the manna dew, which sustained and nourished my firmness of purpose. Nicole vetted the early proofs: thanks to her I made major improvements to comprehensibility and readability. With the enthusiasm of the convert, she works tirelessly to publicize the life-saving knowledge contained in these pages. With her French background, Nicole is an enthusiastic cook. She has delighted in developing ways of preparing delicious food in conformity with the Savanna Model. The reader will find a sample of these recipes in Appendix B (page 127).

This book would not have been possible without the confidence of my publisher, Rudy Shur, of Square One Publishers. In his words, "You have a great rough diamond, we have to release the brilliant stone inside." Thanks to his patient guidance, we transformed the ugly duckling into a swan. Thanks also to my editor, Caroline Smith, who shaped the final drafts and refrained from excising too many of my flights of fancy.

I am indebted to the many expert reviewers whose opinions, encouragement, and advice have improved the relevance, usefulness, and scientific accuracy of the text: Rita Stec, MD, president of the Walter T. Stec Memorial Foundation of Indian Wells, California; Elber S. Camacho, MD, medical director of the Comprehensive Cancer Center, in Palm Springs; Dr. Günter Nöll, of Vienna, Austria, biochemist and authority on edible wild plants; and Caroline Mansfield, ND, director of The Naturopathic Clinic, in London. If, in spite of their efforts, there remain any deficiencies or differences of opinion, then these are mine alone.

Many visionaries helped me on my way in the early days: Christopher Brown, MD, who wrote the excellent foreword to my first book, Joe Schuchert of Kelso Corporation who, with Emmanuel Kampouris as chairman of American Standard, brought my ideas to their workforce, and Steven Gundry, MD, Medical Director of The International Heart Institute of Palm Springs. Many readers and followers have encouraged me with their enthusiasm over the years. It is invidious to single out any one of them. However, I must mention Dr. James Melton, visionary and speaker, for his sage guidance—and Frédéric and Jeanne Bouvet who, persuaded from the very earliest days (some eighteen years ago), produced the first Bond Effect child, Alexandre (and subsequently Diane), using my precepts all the way from inception, through pregnancy to upbringing.

If you are one of the many meritorious contributors whom it has not been possible to cite, just know that you are, like Henry V's unsung heroes, "freshly remember'd" and that your influence lives on in this work. To all of you, and to all of those as yet unsung, my heartfelt thanks.

Introduction

Many people seem to think that nothing can influence their state of health—that it's just like a ticket in the lottery. They do not realize that it is optional, and that the way we eat and lead our lives will decide how we will end up!

Recent studies suggest that each of us has the capacity to live for 100 years, fully functioning to the very end.[1] But that is not happening in today's world. Instead, the average American man will live for 76.4 years and the average woman for 81.2 years.[2] And worse yet, they will spend, on average, the last eight years of life disabled.

Paleo in a Nutshell is going to show you that it doesn't have to be like this! We can take control of our lives and live in harmony the way nature intended—and, by doing so, maximize our lifespan.

What do we need to do? Let me give you an idea: Even a child knows that if you put a cat, a canary, and birdseed in a cage, the cat eats the canary, not the birdseed. We accept, without doubt, the principle that cats and canaries eat differently. Yet we naively think we can feed ourselves—and our kids—*anything*. Many researchers and consumers now know that this is totally wrong and that there is a special feeding pattern for us humans, too.

But the realization does not stop there. Just as zoos now recognize that it is vital for an animal's health that it live the uncaged *lifestyle* that is right for its species, so we now recognize that it is vital for human health to live the *lifestyle* that is right for our species.

A new science explores this fascinating subject: "Evolutionary Lifestyle Anthropology." That is a bit of a mouthful, so we will call it simply "Paleo Lifestyle," so called after the way of life forged in humanity's crucible during the Paleolithic era. This will be explained further in Part 1, "The Paleo Lifestyle."

"The Paleo Lifestyle" is the spellbinding story about what it means to be human, in lifestyle terms. It provides an extraordinarily powerful understanding of how, by living in harmony with the way our bodies are designed, we can rejoice in the best possible health and relish the prospect of a long life.

In this book, we focus on the main aspects of our lifestyle that *mismatch* the way nature designed us. In particular, the food we currently eat is a major cul-

1

prit, but it is followed by other factors too, including physical activity, stress, environment, sunshine, and sleep patterns. An important lesson of this book is that it is not enough to rectify just one of these factors; we have to get *all* the pieces in place.

With regard to feeding patterns, we accept that lions and gorillas have bodies, digestive systems, feeding patterns, and *lifestyles* that are adapted to the environment in which they live. Lions, who live by catching and eating fleet-footed antelope, have razor-sharp claws, needle teeth, and powerful stomach acids. Gorillas, who live by chomping through vast quantities of vegetation, have massive molars and long colons. Lions' bodies are designed to work on the food that lions eat and gorillas' bodies are designed to work on the food that gorillas eat. Yet we imagine, incorrectly, that humans are made to eat anything. The digestive systems we have and the food our ancestors ate millions of years prior to the development of agriculture say otherwise.

What feeding environment are human bodies designed for? Nutritional anthropology shows that there is a very precise specification for the human diet, developed by our human ancestors over millennia, and that our bodies are designed to work according to those instructions and no others. It is an adventure story—stretching across the globe and into the distant past—to discover what humans were designed to eat.

THE PAST IS THE FUTURE

Modern-day humans have changed very little, genetically speaking, and we are still living with bodies and *mentalities* that nature designed for us to thrive in that far-off time. But we are also living with hundreds of lifestyle diseases that our ancestors never experienced. I believe the blame for the emergence of these sicknesses lies with the poor diet and passive lifestyle that we have adopted over the years. Examining our ancestors' way of life provides powerful clues to how we should be living today. These remarkable insights show how, in many surprising and unsuspected ways, we can make critical, life-transforming adjustments. The way humans have been eating and living for many thousands of years has not been ideal. In this book, you will learn how we discovered this and come to understand what you can do to improve and enrich your own life right now.

Our first goal is to open your mind to a whole new way of thinking about the lifestyle that your body needs. Once this reality is accepted, we can move forward to learning how to practice this way of living in today's world. The news is good—we live in a society where we can *take control* for ourselves. For example, today we have a huge variety and abundance of food available from all corners of the globe at any time of the year—we just have to learn how to choose wisely. We can take charge of other aspects, too: With our heightened awareness, we can introduce more physical activity into our lives; we can switch off the electronic devices in the evening and get an early night's sleep; we can actively seek out both the daylight every morning and also the sunshine when we can; we can organize our lives to eliminate avoidable modern-day stressors; and, with thoughtful planning, create a harmonious environment which, by emulating our ancestral landscapes, gives us feelings of reassurance and contentment.

One of the most troubling aspects of our busy lives is the constant bombardment of conflicting messages directed at us by the health and food industries. In this book, we show you the way to peace of mind. The insights of the Paleo lifestyle empower you to judge for yourself. They bring clarity to the confusion and allow you to select with confidence which claims to accept and which to reject. After all, our ancestors knew they were living in a dangerous, treacherous, and unpredictable jungle. They had the skills to survive: They knew how to circumvent a hungry leopard and which mushrooms were poisonous. This book teaches you the skills to survive in today's "supermarket jungle."

The insights of the Paleo lifestyle get at the root causes of the "diseases of civilization": Cancer, heart disease, stroke, diabetes, obesity, arthritis, osteoporosis, Alzheimer's disease, and many more. These diseases are not inevitable; they are optional. These are lifestyle diseases that can be avoided and, if already present, can be stalled and even put into remission. By understanding the principles of Paleo lifestyle and living in accordance with our naturally adapted origins, you can improve your health to be better able to combat any disease and live longer. Your body will find its natural ideal weight, either losing or gaining according to its needs. Instead of losing yourself in the sweeping current of life and circumstance, you will be able to *take control* of your lifestyle habits and thus your life.

These are powerful claims, but as a scientist, I am not given to flights of fancy or guesswork. All the information in this book is based on evidence-driven science. These insights are new, because the various pieces of the puzzle have only recently been put together. For example, peering deep into our DNA is one of the exciting new tools for unlocking the secrets of our genetic heritage. And there are many other fields that are yielding fascinating new insights about how human beings are "designed" to live. This book gathers this scattered, cutting-edge information and synthesizes it into a coherent whole.

But this is not just theory—the ideas work. Over the past two decades, thousands of individuals have been empowered by this information. I have personally worked with many of them to understand the nature of disease, to take control of their eating habits, and to help them live a healthier lifestyle. Many people's lives have been transformed by the insights of the Paleo lifestyle and its handmaiden, Nutritional Anthropology.

THE JOURNEY AHEAD

Part I of this book explains the Paleo lifestyle—how we know what it means to be a human being in lifestyle terms. We highlight the consequences of our divergence from the ideal eating pattern. This part of the book deals with how, as humans, we moved away from our naturally adapted environment, feeding patterns, and lifestyle, and looks at the science supporting our claims. Then, based on these insights, we develop an "Owner's Manual" for how we should be living and feeding ourselves and show you how to put it into action today.

Chapter 1, "Origin and Main Features," describes the remarkable discoveries about human origins, where we come from, and the lifestyle which our ancestral heritage designed for us. It goes on to describe the kinds of foodstuffs that our bodies are designed to eat and the ones that are a mismatch with our ancestral past.

Chapter 2, "Living the Way Nature Intended," describes the main factors of lifestyle which affect us today and compares them with the way they would be in a state of nature. These factors include feeding patterns, physical activity, stress and social environment, nourishment by sunshine, and sleeping patterns.

Chapter 3, "How Did it Go Wrong?,"describes how, over the millennia, more and more new food group interlopers have become part of the modern diet. We explain how they undermine our optimum health in a wide variety of ways, many of them sneaky. It goes on to describe the basic specifications for an ideal food intake in the modern world.

Part II begins with "The Owner's Manual," which summarizes the various aspects of lifestyle and how to harmonize them in a way which our bodies and mentalities recognize. In order to help you make wise food choices, the feeding pattern section grades modern foods according to how well they conform to the Paleo template.

The second chapter in Part II, "Adopting the Paleo Feeding Pattern," is a practical guide to preparing food on a daily basis, for all kinds of consumers from children to the elderly, and for those with special dietary requirements such as vegans and vegetarians. It suggests ways of adopting the Paleo way of eating in three easy stages and gives ideas for the various meals of the day, from breakfast to supper.

The Conclusion, "Healthy Lifespan and the Best of Both Worlds," describes how we can have the best of both worlds: Avoiding the lifestyle diseases of modern societies and avoiding the vicissitudes of life that carried off our forager ancestors. We show how we can aim to not only have a long lifespan, but one that is a *healthy* lifespan right to the end. It is not normal to be sick in old age!

The book concludes with two appendices. The first, "Population Studies Supporting the Paleo Lifestyle," explores a vital source of information: The effect different lifestyles have on health and lifespan as practiced by different populations around the world. This is an important piece of scientific evidence to support the Paleo way of living, but there is much more. This book cuts to the chase on the Paleo lifestyle and does not go into great detail of the scientific evidence. For those who would like to get deep into the scientific background to the Paleo lifestyle, please see my book, *Deadly Harvest*.

Appendix B features Paleo-conforming recipes. Eating the Paleo way can be kept very simple, just by cooking and preparing generic foodstuffs. However, it is also quite possible to produce delicious Paleo-conforming gourmet meals that would please and surprise any dinner guest. In this appendix we include some sample recipes extracted from Nicole Bond's cookbook, *Paleo Harvest.*

This book's fusion of healthy eating with healthy thinking could not be more important, dealing as it does with the absolute fundamentals of human nature. In this guide, you have a focused road map for a trouble-free lifestyle and bodily and mental nutrition. It will be a relief to be clear about where you have to go, and you'll feel better about yourself for taking control of your destiny.

You will find the secret to what it means to be a human being living in close connection with our natural lifestyle. Everyone can use these ideas to enhance his image, inside and out. This book contains the easy-to-learn skills of how to harmonize your life with human genetic programming. We can make adjustments to our ways of eating, our ways of thinking, and our lifestyles so that they coincide as closely as possible with our inherited natural traits. These are the keys to a long, healthy, and harmonious life.

PART I

The Paleo Lifestyle

1.

Origin and Main Features

Being a World War II baby, I spent the first fifteen years of my life on food rations. It is said that we are the "lucky" generation: Many unhealthy foods like sugar, bacon, pork, beef, milk, butter, fat, cakes, and even bread were strictly rationed. Meanwhile, we could eat as much as we liked of cabbage, onions, and turnips!

Be that as it may, the closest I have come to needing hospitalization in my life was when I lived for many years in tropical Africa. One day, back in the 1960s, out in the bush, I got blood poisoning. If that had happened only twenty years earlier, it could have killed me. But I just went along to the local field hospital and, with one massive shot of penicillin, I was cured. It was the archetypal "magic bullet."

Why do I tell you this? To show you that today we can fix just about everything that nature can throw at us. What is left to fight? Our problem now is not what *nature* does to us—it is what we do to ourselves. They are the self-inflicted diseases, the diseases of lifestyle: Cancer, heart disease, diabetes, osteoporosis, arthritis, dementia, and many more. They are caused by the *mismatch* between the lifestyle that nature designed in our ancient past, and the lifestyle we live today. They are diseases of modern industrial societies—they were virtually unknown in prehistoric times.

This guidebook dives into what we know about our prehistoric ancestors—the foragers and hunter-gatherers who lived in the African savannas—and what they did to go through life without encountering any lifestyle diseases. The theory I propose is that their way of living (which we will call the "Paleo way of life") is how humans were designed by nature to live. The way we live today is far from the Paleo way of life—we work inside all throughout the day, we stay up late, we are not very active, and most of all, we now have access to and consume a multitude of highly processed, refined foods. This guidebook will use the research I have gathered to make the argument that we should eat a diet as close as possible to that of the foragers in order for us to live longer, healthier lives.

THE BENEFITS OF THE PALEO LIFESTYLE

We now know that when you adopt the Paleo way of life, you immediately improve your chances of never getting:

- Cancer
- Heart disease
- Artery disease (Arteriosclerosis)
- Diabetes
- Osteoporosis

- Arthritis
- Alzheimer's disease
- Obesity
- Inflammatory bowel diseases
- Mood disorders

If you already have one or more of these conditions, the Paleo lifestyle can give you the best chance of stabilizing them or even putting them into remission.

The Paleo lifestyle, as we will explore in this guide, is a way of living as nature intended. Every aspect of our lifestyles—our diets, activity levels, sleeping patterns, familial relations—has been genetically programmed into us. However, things have changed over the millions of years that our ancestors have existed, and we have gotten so far away from our ideal lifestyles that the diseases mentioned above are considered commonplace.

You will be forgiven some skepticism at this point. These are some pretty tall promises. So, read on; we think the facts of the Paleo lifestyle will overcome any uncertainty.

SCIENCE ENDORSES THE HUNTER-GATHERER

I have been researching ancient lifestyle patterns for decades, and my first publications came out in the 1990s. (See "Supplemental Research" on page 11.) The Paleo lifestyle is one for which us humans are *genetically programmed.*

We find that what we know about the ancestral lifestyle dovetails perfectly with the conclusions of scientific studies of what we know works with our biology, biochemistry, digestive systems, and even our mentalities.

The conclusion: Our "primitive" ancestors lived in harmony with the way the human body is best designed. Today, we've strayed alarmingly far from this lifestyle—the one that's natural for our species. Today, most of our food supply is "novelty" food, newfangled concoctions introduced only in the last 11,000 years. Today, our lives are lived in ways which starve us of the right kind of physical activity, of enough sunshine, of good sleep, and which trigger stress reactions in ways that our nerves were never designed to handle.

So what is this "naturally adapted" lifestyle? It was one that made us "fit for purpose" in our ancestral homeland. To understand what it is, we have to go back to our origins.

Supplemental Research

For those curious, my appraisals and research have examined the following:

- The human digestive system and how it is designed to work.

- Human body chemistry and how it is designed to work.

- Species like gorillas and chimps with bodies similar to ours.

- Forensic archaeology—analysis of ancient bone composition, revealing how our ancestors lived and nourished themselves.

- Population studies—why some peoples like the Cretans and Okinawans are healthier and live longer. (See Appendix A on page 117.)

- Clinical trials—testing sample groups for the medical effects of living different ways.

- Anthropology—how ancient and contemporary hunter-gatherers live.

- Reverse engineering—what we know works for us today.

- Tooth morphology, tooth wear, and tooth plaque.

- Optimal foraging strategy—how humans made best use of the feeding opportunities open to them by a savanna lifestyle.

- Tool marks on animal bones, revealing the kinds of animals humans hunted and ate.

See Resources on page 146 for more information.

Our Origins and our Homeland

Since the 1960s, the evidence piled up about our African origins until the clincher came from a quite unexpected quarter—the study of genetics.

Thanks to studies of DNA, we now know that everyone on the *planet* is descended from a small group of people who lived just 60,000 years ago (2,000 generations ago) in the savannas of the Great Rift Valley of East Africa.

At that time, humans and their ancestral species had lived there for millions of years. They used simple stone tools and, for this reason, this immense period of time is called "Paleolithic," from the Greek words for "Old" and "Stone"— Old Stone Age.

The Meaning of Paleo

The Paleolithic Age is how we get the word "Paleo." It has become the byword for living the way I discuss in this guide and have been talking about for over twenty years. However, it has also become a popular term that is misused by food manufacturers for profit. (See "Be Wary of the 'Paleo' Label" inset below.)

Moreover, and this is crucial, we know that we are all still living with bodies and brains designed for life in the savannas. Sure, we've changed a bit on the outside since then, but we are still the same 60,000 year-old model underneath. Above all, we are still tropical creatures—it's not for nothing that we want to come and live in places with sunshine and palm trees! We still have the same physiology, the same digestive system, the same biochemistry, and the same *mentalities* as for life back then.

THE HUMAN TIMELINE

If our homeland (our "Garden of Eden") is in the African savannas, how did we fill up the rest of the world?

We can now piece together what happened. Over a period of a million years, successive waves of humanlike creatures overflowed out of Africa to populate most of the Old World. They had brains about half the size of ours, but walked upright and had many humanlike traits. They have been broadly called *Homo erectus*, of which the Neanderthals were just one branch. Then, about 200,000 years ago, a radical thing happened: A new breed of *Homo erectus* arose in East Africa—our own ancestor, *Homo sapiens*.

Be Wary of the "Paleo" Label

The name "Paleo" is often hijacked to promote diets which bear little or no resemblance to the real thing. For example, there is a misconception that humans ate mammoth meat by the hundredweight, and so we should all be eating fatty bacon and pork chops by the bucketful. Wrong!

Another misconception is to imagine that ancient grains (e.g., einkorn and emmer wheat) are somehow forager food and therefore are allowable in the Paleo diet—they are not! Indeed, they were the first grains to be farmed. Similarly, pseudo grains like quinoa and amaranth are just that: Pseudo grains, with all the drawbacks of true grains. Avoid!

Others, more unscrupulous, carelessly attach the word "Paleo" simply to sell manufactured foodstuffs, even though they bear no resemblance to a true Paleo food—keep your wits about you and avoid!

In this work we deal with the *authentic* Paleo lifestyle—and nothing else.

Homo sapiens were brainier, more agile, more inventive, but more lightly built than *Homo erectus*. They were successful in their ability to survive and to multiply. However, to feed themselves, they needed around 200 square miles of living space per band of fifty people. So, in their turn, from about 75,000 to 60,000 years ago, they overflowed in waves out of Africa into Australia, Asia, Europe, and finally the Americas (see Figure 1.1 on the following page).

So that is the key to the question. What is this savanna lifestyle that has shaped us humans? Now, after years of research, we have been able to build up a complete picture of what life was like for our Paleolithic ancestors.

Life on the Savannas

Our ancestors lived in groups of some forty to fifty people—about nine or ten families. They had a territory of about 200 square miles within which they wandered. They camped for a while in one place and, when they were done there, they walked, old people and toddlers included, 10 to 15 miles to the next campsite.

Every day, the women went off foraging in a group, carrying toddlers on their backs. For safety, they stayed in contact with each other by keeping up a stream of chatter called "rapport talk." If one of them stopped hearing the chatter, she would get uneasy and link up with the group again. After three or four hours, the women came back with some 15 to 25 lbs (7 to 10 kg) of the food they had collected.

The men would go off on their own: Trapping, scavenging, or occasionally hunting. They provided about 15 percent of the food supply, and it was almost entirely animal matter and some honey. Even though it was not a high proportion of the total amount of food, their contribution was high-status "trophy food." Back at the camp, the men would sit around a campfire and recount their exploits of the day. This is known as "report talk."

Both men and women would eat some of what they collected as they went along, but the major part they would bring back to the camp—a procedure called "central place provisioning." Mostly they shared with the other members of the family but, if there was enough left over, they would share with other members of the band, either to settle debts or to create reciprocal obligations.

Plant Food and Animal Food Ratio

All together, people ate about 2.5 lbs plant food (of a particular kind) and 8 to 12 oz animal food per day. This gives a ratio of about 75 percent plant food to about 25 percent animal matter. As we shall see later, this ratio is quite important.

Fire and Cooking

Homo sapiens knew all about fire—indeed, his ancestral species *Homo erectus* had discovered how to master fire some 1 million years ago. So foragers routinely roasted foods in the embers of the fire. This would include tubers, nuts, and

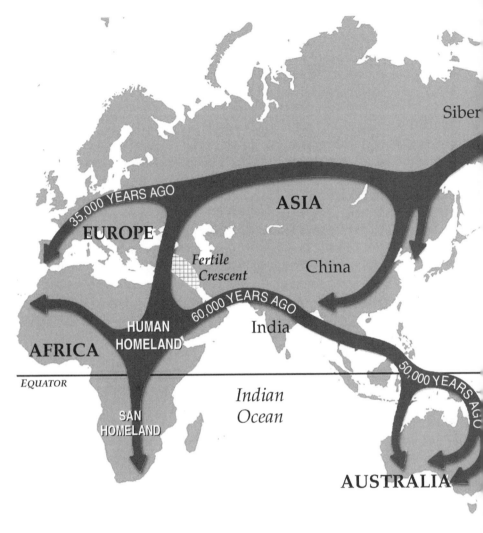

Figure 1.1. Human Migration Out of Africa.

various parts of the animal carcass. Some authorities believe that cooking (roasting) of some foods was a necessary condition for *Homo sapiens* to evolve. At any rate, there is no basis for the belief that humans should be eating a totally raw food diet.

But roasting was just about the only cooking method available to foragers— no boiling, steaming, or sautéing for them! However, on occasion, they would bury a carcass with embers under a mound of earth and slow cook it that way.

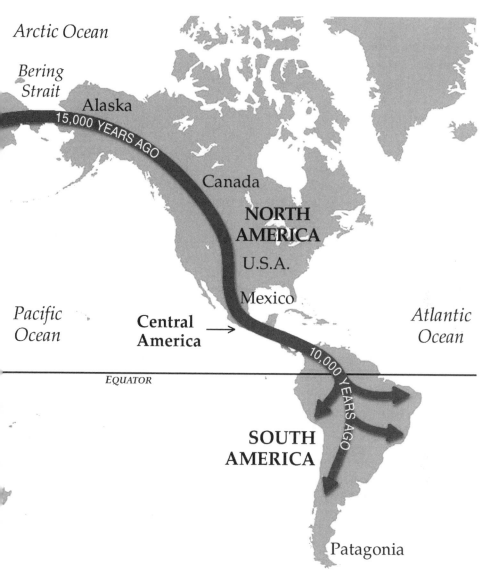

Physical Activity

On average, women walked some 3 to 4 miles every day, carrying loads most of the time. The men would walk and run some 7 to 8 miles every day. As we shall see later, if this was the physical activity pattern for men and women down through the eons, then the body came to rely on it being there—and if it is not there, things go wrong.

This went on down the seasons, down the centuries, down the millennia. At that time, their bodies were basically in equilibrium with their environment.

What Was Their Health Like?

Even today there are peoples, like the San Bushmen of Southern Africa, who still live this way. What is their health like?

The San are in excellent health by any terms, let alone under the arduous conditions in which they live. Their old people live to a venerable yet healthy old age, in good shape right to the end. This is an important lesson for us all. It is not normal to be decrepit in old age. We are meant to be fit for purpose right to the end—and if you can't walk those 12 miles to the next campsite, you are left for dead!

Predictably, the San do not suffer from obesity or the diseases it causes. Diabetes is unknown. They have low levels of phospholipids and triglycerides (types of fat molecules). Especially significant, they have one of the lowest cholesterol levels in the world: Total cholesterol levels for all age groups are around 120 mg/dL, compared with about 200 mg/dL in Westerners. This is in spite of them eating *more* cholesterol than the typical Westerner! How can this be? The answer is that our dysfunctional Western lifestyle irritates our bodies into making cholesterol, even when it is not needed. We shall see later how this happens.

The diet is very low in fats of all kinds, and the types of fats are healthier. Compared with Westerners, the San have a much higher percentage of omega-3 fat (26 percent compared with 9 percent) and a lower percentage of omega-6 fat (34 percent to 40 percent). This is not surprising: In contrast to Westerners, the San are eating a diet that contains roughly equal amounts of omega-3 and omega-6 fats. The main sources of fats for the San are nuts and wild creatures, both of which have very different fatty acid profiles to the foods habitually consumed in the West. (See Chapter 3 for more information about these fatty acids.)

There is no sign of coronary heart disease, atherosclerosis, or thrombosis. Researchers have found no case of varicose veins, piles, or hernias. No cases of cancer or osteoporosis have been seen either. Average blood pressure is a low 120/75 and it does not increase with age; not a single case was found of high blood pressure.[1]

Hearing tests on ten elderly Bushmen found that they had perfect hearing.[2] There was little or no earwax and the eardrum could be easily seen. Teeth were also free of caries (cavities). In old age, eyesight still remained excellent for distance. The San received healthy levels of vitamins A, B12, C, and D, folate, thiamine, riboflavin, niacin, iron, calcium, iodine, zinc, copper, and other trace elements.

The human body is designed to manufacture vitamin D from sunlight. The San, like our African Pleistocene ancestors, live in a sunny place and spend all day outdoors, with no clothes on. Their bodies manufacture all the vitamin D they need. Nobody suffers from anemia or protein deficiency. The kidneys are functioning normally on the low-salt diet and are excreting very little salt in the urine. Levels of phosphorus in the urine are very low.

Lactose is a type of sugar found uniquely in milk. It is an aggressive allergen for most adults, although some Caucasians can put up with it. The San, in common with most peoples of the world, are uniformly intolerant of lactose.

In *glucose tolerance* tests, the San had responses that are within the normal, non-diabetic range. Insulin response is slow, as is normal for humans who have virtually no sugars in the diet.

In other words, foragers don't suffer from all the conditions that we rightly call *diseases of civilization*. This opens up a magical possibility—that we can *choose* not to have them!

MAIN FEATURES OF THE PALEO LIFESTYLE

In the subsequent sections, we will take a look at the main features of the Paleo lifestyle, as follows:

- Feeding patterns and food supply
- Sunshine and sunlight
- Sleeping patterns
- Physical activity
- Stress

Feeding Patterns and Food Supply

Since few of the foods that foragers ate in our ancient past are available to us today, we have to identify the *basic characteristics* of the food supply and emulate it in today's world. The good news is that it is easily done once you have mastered the basic ideas.

These are the kinds of foods that constituted our ancestral diet:

Plant food	Animal matter
• Bulbs and tubers	• Eggs
• Tree nuts	• Mammal meat and offal (organ)
• Fruits and berries	• Birds
• Edible leaves and stalks	• Fish, shellfish
• Funguses and mushrooms	• Tortoises, turtles
• Gourds and squashes	• Insects, caterpillars, locusts
• Flowers	• Reptiles—snakes and lizards
• Honey	• Amphibians (e.g., frogs)

Imitating the Specification

Don't be put off by some of the bizarre foods. We are *not* saying you will have to start eating locusts, turtles, and frogs! (Although many societies from Africa to Asia do.) No—what we are saying is that we need to find everyday foods which have the same specification in our own supermarkets. And the good news it is perfectly possible—even easy.

On the other hand, it is interesting to note which everyday foods are *not* on the list. Most obviously, there are no cereals (like wheat and barley), no legumes (like beans and lentils), and no dairy (like milk, yogurt, and cheese). As we shall see, they are "invasive species" in the modern diet and they contribute hugely to the famous "mismatch," which is making us overweight and sick.

It Helps to Know What We Are Not

You've probably heard that humans are described as "omnivores," meaning "eaters of everything"—as if we were carnivores, herbivores, and all the rest rolled into one. Now, while most of us behave as if that were true, from the standpoint of biology, it really isn't.

We're not designed as carnivores. Natural meat-only eaters, like cats, have teeth designed for tearing. Ours are designed for grinding. Cats have different digestive tracts, with powerful gastric juices and protein digestion enzymes. We have long digestive tracts, with weaker gastric juices and enzymes. Ours is a tract which, on a wholly meat diet, becomes a lengthy toxic sewer. Evidence suggests that our ancient ancestors' diet did include some 25 percent animal matter. But—and this is important—much of it was largely the kinds of animals you could catch with your bare hands (see list on page 17). It definitely was not our modern fatty farm meat.

We're not designed as herbivores. Herbivores are grass-eaters, like cattle and sheep. They have several stomachs and symbiotic bacteria to help them draw nutrition from grass and straw. We, obviously, are a couple of stomachs short. Even if humans do try to live on grass, they starve.

We're not designed as lactivores. Lactivores are creatures that live on a diet of milk. A human baby is a lactivore, but only for around the first three years of life. Remember that nursery rhyme about curds and whey? A baby's body manufactures enzymes that curdle the milk, separate the curds from the whey, and digest it all quite nicely. But the body stops making these enzymes at around three years of age. After that, an indigestible clump of goo wends its way through your digestive system. Worse than that, most humans on the planet (including the San Bushmen) no longer secrete the enzyme *lactase* to digest the milk's cargo of *lactose*. As we will see later, lactose is a mischief-maker in a wide range of diseases and ailments.

We're not designed as granivores. These are the grain and cereal eaters, like chickens. They have crops as well as stomachs and swallow stones to grind the seeds they eat. Humans do not. *We cannot digest raw cereals.* They have to be preprocessed first, like breakfast cereals, or cooked, like bread, pasta, or cakes. This is a big topic and we will see in Chapter 3 why grains are best avoided.

If We Are Not Omnivores, What Kind of Creature Are We?

We are first and foremost a salad-fruit-plant eater, with some animal matter thrown in. That's what we are by design, if not by habit. Our body design takes it for granted that we will eat salads, fruits, and vegetables in large quantities every day. So let's just see what that means exactly.

Plant Food Specification

The plant food eaten by our ancestors was of a particular kind. It was:

- Alkalizing.
- Rich in micronutrients.
- Rich in fiber—soluble, insoluble, and downright indigestible "roughage."
- Low in sodium, rich in potassium.
- Low-glycemic and low-insulinemic (i.e., doesn't give sharp blood sugar spikes or insulin spikes).

Alkalizing

When the appropriate food is digested and passes into the body, it has an alkalizing effect on the body fluids. The human body is designed on the basis that the diet will be slightly alkalizing overall. In forager diets, the alkalizing plants are counterbalanced—almost—by the animal protein, which is acidifying.

As we saw earlier, the *ratio* of plant food to animal matter is about 75 percent to 25 percent by weight. This ratio leads to the slightly alkalizing diet that we need. However, today, we have a problem: We eat plants that are *not* alkalizing. Notably, these are starches like grains (breakfast cereals, pasta, pizza, breads, cakes, and pastry) and potato (boiled, French fried, and baked). In fact, we eat these in such huge quantities that the Western diet is relentlessly *acidic*.

This puts tremendous stresses on the body's biochemistry and organs. A chronically acidic diet:

- Weakens bones by dragging out calcium to neutralize the acid.
- Irritates the kidneys into leaking calcium.
- Leads to kidney stones.
- Undermines the health of the pancreas, the lymphatic system, the thyroid, and the liver.

So these are some of the reasons why grains and potatoes are not human food.

Micronutrients

The forager plant food was rich in micronutrients. And when we talk about micronutrients, it's not just vitamins and minerals, but also the tens of thousands of *bioflavonoids, phenols, carotenoids,* and many more.

Our modern diets are chronically *deficient* in micronutrients—and it is not due to depleted soils or whatnot. It is due to eating foods that, by their very nature, are poor in micronutrients. What are these foods? None other than starches like potato and grains (cereals). By eating these foods in vast quantities, we starve our bodies of micronutrients.

Many studies show that it is futile to try to make up the deficiency with supplements. There is something about getting micronutrients in food: They work together in ways that we do not understand and probably never will. It is like an orchestra where all the players have to be working together in harmony for them to be effective.

Fiber

Forager plant food was rich in fiber of all kinds: Soluble, insoluble, and downright indigestible. These indigestible fibers, mainly from forager tubers, are particularly intriguing. They are stringy and composed of materials like cellulose. They pass straight through the digestive tract completely unchanged. There is nothing like them in the modern food supply; yet, since they were all-pervasive in our ancient ancestors' lives, they probably performed a useful function.

The San consumed a high-fiber diet and their plant matter was naturally very fibrous. Remarkably, it has been possible to examine 11,000-year-old fossilized forager feces. It showed that our ancestors were consuming 130 g per day of plant fibers, much of them the indigestible fibers discussed above. But we don't have to go back to our ancient past: In the 1970s Dr. Denis Burkitt, with his own observations,[3] reported that rural Africans passed stool that was up to five times greater by mass; had intestinal transit times that were more than twice as fast; and ate three to seven times more dietary fiber than their Western counterparts (60–140 g versus 20 g).[4] The average American only consumes about 13 g per day, which is sharply under even the modest target set by various health authorities of around 30 g per day.

The colon is a hive of activity—in hundreds of ways, it affects the health of the whole body. Our guts are also the scene of intense warfare between "friendly" organisms and unfriendly ones. We can be reasonably sure that the San's colons functioned as nature intended. All is not well with the way we eat today. We are sending down residues that our intestines do not recognize and that promote malevolent gut flora. Passage through the intestines is slow and consists of foods that destroy the delicate gut wall and undermine the immune system.

Low in Sodium, Rich in Potassium

Our Paleolithic environment contained no free salt. The only sodium was what was intrinsic to the food they ate. Our ancestors had a low sodium intake. However, they had a high potassium intake—such that their ratio between sodium and potassium was about 1:5. It turns out that this is a critical ratio in human biochemistry. But today, we have reversed this ratio to be about 5:1 sodium to potassium. This happens because, yes, we eat so many foods—mainly processed—that are full of sodium. (Did you know that cornflakes have more salt in them than seawater does?) But our high sodium intake ratio also happens because of the absence of potassium-bearing foods; these are the salads, vegetables, and fruits that our ancient past programmed us to eat.

This imbalance has numerous consequences:

- It raises blood pressure in many people.

- It inflames and scars arteries.

- Sodium is a calcium "antagonist"—the more sodium you take in, the less calcium you absorb.

- It stops cells from excreting sodium waste from within the cell. (Every cell has to pump sodium out against a sodium gradient in the surrounding fluids. When we increase the sodium gradient many-fold, then the pumping mechanism cannot cope; the cell malfunctions or dies.)

Low-Glycemic and Low-Insulinemic

Nature designed us humans to work on a "low-glycemic" diet. That is, our diet should not give us harmful blood sugar spikes. But today, we do the opposite. Chances are, you are giving yourself a rollercoaster of sharp blood sugar spikes several times a day. Why might this be a problem?

First, abnormally high blood glucose levels create problems directly. For example, it can cause the death of nerve endings, leading to blindness, death of kidney tissue, and fatty liver. Worse, they feed cancers!

Back in the 1980s, Dr. David Jenkins devised the concept of the Glycemic Index—a measure of how likely a given food will give a blood sugar spike. The closer it is to 100, the worse it is. Here are some examples.

EXAMPLES OF GLYCEMIC INDEXES					
BAD		**BORDERLINE**		**FAVORABLE**	
Corn flakes	85	Dates, raisins	60	Raspberries	25
Baked potato	85	Rice, brown	55	Walnuts	15
Bread	70	Spaghetti	45	Tomato	15
Sugar	65	Banana (unripe)	40	Lettuce	15

Second, to deal with the glucose spikes, the body produces spikes of insulin. Insulin is a powerful hormone which can be like a bull in a china shop, knocking over the furniture. It disrupts our biochemistry in many ways: We are familiar with diabetes and metabolic syndrome, but there are several other conditions too.

Because insulin is a powerful hormone which directs the production of many other hormones, when insulin is dysfunctional, it creates havoc with many other processes.

I like to think about it as an iceberg: All you see are isolated ailments above the surface, but they are all linked underneath by the lurking menace of hyper-insulinemia—which you can't see or feel and which makes it all the more dangerous.

So insulin depresses the immune system (allowing cancers to flourish), depresses bone building, increases histamine, depresses mood, increases blood clotting and plaque formation, and so on. It is one of the main reasons why we have high cholesterol levels, and it is even a factor in acne!

Our Western diet is high-insulinemic, so right here we see how it is responsible for a lot of mischief. Foragers often combat high insulin levels by allowing themselves to feel hungry several times a day. This practice releases glucagon, a hormone that undoes damage from insulin. In contrast, we often find ourselves eating all throughout the day—even when we are not hungry. (See inset "The Importance of Feeling Hungry," page 23.)

Let's look at typical insulin indexes, because there are some surprises.

SOME INSULIN INDEXES		
FOODS	INSULIN RESPONSE	INSULIN INDEX
Mars bar	High	122
Potatoes	High	121
Beans, baked	High	120
Yogurt, fruit	High	115
Bread, white	High	100
Fish	Normal	59
Beef	Normal	51
Eggs	Normal	31

"An Insulin Index of Foods," S.H. Holt et al., 1997.[5]

As we might expect, the high-glycemic foods (such as bread and potatoes) produce a strong insulin response. But baked beans may be a surprise for you—and who would have suspected that of yogurt? Meanwhile, the insulin reaction to protein-rich foods like fish and eggs is "normal."

There are two lessons:

- Highly refined bakery and snack products give abnormal insulin reactions

- Sugars/starches and proteins provoke different insulin reactions. When sugar/starch is combined with protein, the insulin level is raised many times more than the two separate reactions combined.

The conclusion is that the Western staples, bread and potato, are among the most insulin-raising of foods. Similarly, the highly refined bakery products and snack foods induced substantially more insulin secretion than other test foods. As we shall see, none of these, including yogurt, is either healthy or a human food.

Our Living Gut

Our bodies are built on the assumption that a certain kind of biomass will be living in our colons. It lives in symbiotic relationship with the rest of our body. This biomass is highly active. It cross-talks with the immune system—lymphocytes do not mature properly if they do not get the right signals from "good" bacteria

The Importance of Feeling Hungry

One of the most important feeding patterns of the foragers is to induce hunger from time to time. The typical forager man is skinny—his body fat percentage will be around 8 percent with a body mass index (BMI) of 18. Women would have around 12 percent body fat. All the evidence points to the fact that this is the way to be: Low body fat is best for health and long life.

Being hungry several times a day:

- Contributes to weight loss and low body fat percentage.

- Causes the body to secrete the hormone glucagon. Glucagon is the antidote to insulin and it will undo mischief that insulin might have done.

- Quenches degenerative disease.

- Extends lifespan (at least in non-human creatures).

- Quenches inflammation and oxidative stress.

We are not saying that you have to be as skinny as a forager, but to feel a little hungry for an hour before the next meal. Life is not fair in these days of abundant food supply—foragers would go searching for food and might or might not be successful, while today we open the fridge door and are successful 100 percent of the time!

on the colon wall. It nourishes the gut micro-villi, and it produces biochemical compounds like butyric acid and propionic acid, which pass through the gut wall to nourish the immune system. In other words, it should be like an herb garden down there.

But for most of us, it is the opposite: Our colons are like toxic sewers, undermining our health in many ways. We have overgrowth of "bad" bacteria. They are sulfur-reducing bacteria, and they generate hydrogen sulfide and sulfuric acid. Just from this alone, they give rise to all kinds of bowel disease, including ulcerative colitis, irritable bowel, and cancer. Worse, these bacteria do not cross-talk with the immune system, and so do not help it develop properly. They are sneaky: They loosen the tight junctions of the colon wall and allow themselves, bad funguses like Candida, and food particles to invade the blood stream and create mischief. Finally, they smell bad!

In other respects, our diet is deficient in the volume and quality of plant residue that the colon expects. The result is slow transit times, constipation, and diverticulosis.

Researchers are painstakingly identifying connections between many pathologies and poor flora profile, or *dysbiosis*. Here are some of them:

- Inflammation and auto-immune diseases.[6,7]
- Type 1 diabetes.[8]
- Multiple sclerosis.[9,10,11]
- Bone building.[12,13]
- Cystitis, bladder irritation and pelvic pain.[14]
- Allergies through poor bacterial diversity.[15]
- Stress, upsetting gut bacteria and immune response.[16]
- Behavior, mood, and the brain.[17]
- Serotonin and happiness connection.[18]
- Sloth and anxiety connection.[19]
- Autism, anxiety, and neurotic behaviors.[20]
- Cognitive flexibility.[21]
- Toddler temper and gut.[22]
- Metabolic changes, including obesity, type 2 diabetes, atherosclerosis, and non-alcoholic fatty liver disease.[23]
- Microbe diversity decimators, among them antacids, antibiotics, and the diabetes drug metformin.[24,25]
- Obesity.[26]
- Gut bugs and uveitis.[27]

In other words, maintaining a healthy gut profile is essential to preventing or even reversing the above conditions. Later on in this guide, I will explain which foods can help you achieve this balance.

CONCLUSION

Over eighty years ago, author/philosopher and Nobel Prize nominee Aldous Huxley, in his book *Brave New World,* said: "The scientist will prepare the bed on which mankind must lie; and if mankind doesn't fit—well, that will be just too bad for mankind. There will have to be some stretching and a bit of amputation." As Huxley noted, we are living in a highly artificial world. It has come about through the blind workings of runaway science, technology, and economic forces. The result is a world that is not designed to fit with human nature! On the contrary, in so many ways it cuts across our savanna-bred biology and mentality, driving us into stress, neuroses, sickness, and disease.

This book is not about changing the world—it cannot be! But there is hope. We can take back a little control for ourselves by returning to the ways of our ancestors. I believe the way they ate and lived is directly related to the nonexistence of lifestyle diseases in their societies. I will help you draw comparisons between the past and the present in Chapter 2.

2.

Living the Way Nature Intended

n Chapter 1, I outlined the main features of the Paleo lifestyle—feeding patterns, sunshine, sleeping patterns, physical activity, and stress—and went into detail about the first feature, the feeding patterns of our forager ancestors. In Chapter 2, I discuss the environmental aspects of the Paleo lifestyle (sunshine, sleeping patterns, physical activity, and stress) and how they interact with food and feeding patterns to enhance our well-being.

We have seen that, in a state of nature, gut flora perform a vital symbiotic role in our bodies' biochemistry. It is like an auxiliary organ, working away silently in the background, part of a team keeping human bodies healthy.

But we are not in a state of nature. Western lifestyles in particular have degenerated to the point where our gut flora is worse than useless—it is making us sick. The liberal use of antibiotics, mostly for trivial purposes, is compounding the harm by indiscriminately wiping out gut flora wholesale. In so doing it is, probably, damaging an individual's microbiome in ways from which it will never recover.

However, this is no reason to give up. The message throughout this book is that we can stack the deck of cards in our favor. So, the first thing is, yes, if you live and eat the way we say, this will restore a much better floral balance—even if it is not perfect. Second, if it were me, I'd try to restrict the use of antibiotics, those "wonder drugs," to life-saving purposes only.

As for the problem of the extinct bacteria in Western populations, perhaps the time will come when newborns are routinely inoculated—along with whooping cough, measles, and mumps jabs—with forager stool transplants. In sooth such things have been!

ENVIRONMENT

Studies show that we feel most comfortable, *reassured*, when we are living in an environment of open green spaces with abundant vegetation and occasional trees. In other words, a kind of parkland which speaks to something deep in our psyches. It speaks to us of our ancestral savannas—of *home*.

In these conditions, people feel better adjusted mentally. A familiar and comforting environment helps improve ADHD, sociability, mood, recovery in hospital, morale in hospices, and ameliorate Alzheimer's disease. How are these effects achieved? Chronic *inflammation* is a major factor in all of them. Living in an environment in harmony with our psyches *quenches* this harmful inflammation. We even find that patients in hospital wards facing the gardens do better than patients overlooking the car park.

People prefer to work in indoor and outdoor spaces which offer protection at the back and overhead. Lone diners in a restaurant prefer to sit with their backs to the wall, facing the center. Surveys show that people like settings with soft rounded forms and irregular layouts. They especially dislike vast institutional spaces with minimal décor.

Population Density and the Pull of the City

Paleolithic humans had a very low population density. While fifty persons comprising a band of foragers lived in close proximity to each other, the nearest neighboring band would be 20 to 30 miles away. At various times of the year, groups would meet up for a festival. It was the occasion to find mates, trade artifacts, overeat, and have a good time. Even so, those humans did not meet more than a few hundred different people in a lifetime. There is no doubt that, in the wandering band of fifty or so people, life could seem dull compared to the excitement of the festival.

Today, the excitement, anonymity, and opportunities of living in crowded cities operate on our minds like a recreational drug. Most of us have felt the tug-of-war in our lives between the buzz of working in a city during the day, but fleeing to the calm of the leafy green suburbs at the end of the day. It is true, too, that the city can provide an intoxicating mix of stimulation and excitement that was unknown in forager times. It is like a drug, so the trick is to not let it become an addiction. Is there a downside to living in such crowding?

The American ethologist John Calhoun published a pioneering animal study in 1970 and found that crowded female rats had low fertility rates and high rates of miscarriage and death in childbirth; they also had poor nesting and poor parenting behaviors. Male rats had high rates of sexual deviation, homosexuality, aggression, violence, cannibalism, pathological depression, and withdrawal. There were high rates of social disorientation, infanticide, and infant mortality. Calhoun finished his report with the observation that we might advance our understanding "about analogous problems confronting the human species."[1]

Does this have the ring of truth to it? Today's high population densities have put us on a treadmill requiring industrialized, intensive forms of society. Many of us are worn down by congestion, crowds, and lack of time to even think. We dream of lives in closer contact with natural surroundings. There is no doubt that our mentalities are best adapted to much lower population densities. Do follow your instincts if you feel "the call of the wild"—it is natural and good for your psyche, and that of your family, to seek an environment where you are well-adjusted.

Role of Myth, Ritual, and Trance

Primal tribes have traditions where, several times a month, they dance all night to rhythmic drumming until they reach a trance-like state. When they are like this, they feel like they've merged with the universe and made contact with the great unknown. They emerge from this state with a tremendous feeling of having purged emotional tension.

Maybe noisy nightclubs, music festivals, and the like are, in a similar way, fulfilling a deep psychological need. Of course, there are many other ways of chilling out—and, it seems, chill out we must from time to time. That is where meditation, yoga, or just a relaxing soak in a hot bath perform their secret ministry. These modern substitutes have not been compared to the forager way of relaxing, so we do not know if they are as effective—but it seems that they do have a place in our lives.

The Workplace

When we think about our naturally adapted origins, the only work people had was foraging and hunting. Now, think about this: They only spent fifteen to twenty hours a week doing it. Today, we work at least double that.

Secondly, the women doing their foraging felt *fulfilled*. They felt good about collecting for their children and family. Likewise, the men found their work fulfilling: They went off to do battle with nature, using ingenuity, bravery, and subtle skills to bring home the bacon. They felt good about it; it made them feel important and it gave them a sense of identity.

Thirdly, as we saw in "Life on the Savannas" (see page 13), the women would work together and indulge in "rapport talk"; the men would work independently and practiced "report talk." Today's workplaces make no allowances for these ingrained differences in ways of working.

Fourthly, and most importantly, there were *no* employers, *no* employees, and *no* jobs. You wanted something to feed your family? You just got up, wandered into the bush and got started! No one could stop you. You didn't have to hustle for a "job," you didn't have to worry about career; no one had control of your livelihood.

That is where the modern world is at its most dysfunctional. It is very hard to regain control of your livelihood—and even harder to regain control of your time. But we do know that people who do have greatest control over these matters are much better adjusted mentally. Such people might be at the very top of organizations, or just self-employed in any capacity. We also know that in areas with high rates of self-employment, the whole community is better adjusted, too.[2]

The Vital Role of Grandmothers

Not many species have lifespans that cover three generations, so there must be an evolutionary reason why this should be—something about having grandparents around that promotes survival of their genes in their grandchildren. Kirsten Hawkes (department of anthropology, University of Utah) pioneered a now well-accepted explanation: That grandparents—and in particular daughters' grandmothers—played a vital role in the survival of humanity.[3]

Studies show that forager grandmothers contributed more collected food than any other category in the forager band. Moreover, they contributed a high level of childcare, freeing up the mothers to forage in their turn. The conclusion is that without grandmothers, we would have gone extinct. Consequently, evolutionary pressures have wired grandmother's brains to "want to be with the grandchildren." That is, grandmothers are strongly programmed to nurture their grandchildren.

It is a modern tragedy that grandmothers, for the most part, do not play a major—or any—role in bringing up the grandchildren. This creates three sets of stressed-out people: The grandmother, who has a frustrated yearning to be with the grandchildren (and the grandfather, who is stressed because his wife is stressed); the parents, who become twenty-four-hour parenting automatons; and the children, who are stressed because the parents are stressed. This is another example of how, by aligning our life decisions with our savanna-bred natures, we can reduce background stress.

Social Connectedness

The forager band of some fifty people would be a closely-knit community. They are the in-group and they all look out for each other. This is the archetypal extended family. For example, kids can run to anyone in the group if they need help; adults will help out with the kids, even if the kids are not their own.

However, there is more to it than that. Compared to today, this group of people has a higher degree of "social connectedness." That is, they have more links—and stronger links—with the other members of the community. On the other hand, their links to spouse and children are less frenetic than in today's "nuclear family." In the modern world, society has become atomized and the nuclear family has become the norm—but it is against the laws of nature and is unnaturally intense and stressful.

SUNSHINE AND SUNLIGHT

When we look at those foragers—when we think of our evolutionary history— humans spent 365 days a year, stark naked, under a tropical sun. If that was the case for millions of years, we can be sure that our bodies came to depend on it.

And now, because of a totally misplaced fear of melanoma (skin cancer), Westerners are suffering from sunshine deficiency! These are some of the major diseases of which sunshine deprivation is a factor:

- Osteoporosis[4]
- Dementia[5]
- Depression[6]
- Multiple sclerosis (MS)[7,8]

- Diabetes[9]
- Cancer[10,11,12,13,14,15]
- Obesity[16]
- High blood pressure[17]

Indeed, researchers conclude that avoiding the sun is actually as bad for you as smoking. The first thing to know is that sunshine deficiency increases *inflammation*.[18] And inflammation underlies most of these conditions, notably cancers (including leukemia). A second factor is this: Sunshine triggers the release of *nitric oxide*, which helps control blood pressure, cardiovascular disease, and the mood hormone *serotonin*.

And just in case you are concerned about melanoma, it is just as likely to occur on parts of the body that have never seen the sun, like the gums and the soles of the feet. Indeed, melanomas can occur *anywhere*—under the armpits and even the genitals. Moreover, we find that melanoma patients are more likely to make a good recovery if they have *more* sunshine rather than less!

What about the use of sunscreen? This is one of the major health scandals: Using sunscreen switches off the alarm (the burning), but allows the DNA damage—so you are *more* likely to get a skin cancer if you use sunscreen.

But the tide is turning: There has been a vigorous debate in the *British Medical Journal* (BMJ) suggesting that doctors have been overzealous in demonizing sunshine.[19] And more recently, a consortium of the major UK health institutions—including the dermatologists—has recommended that Britons should get out in the midday sun without sunscreen for at least ten minutes.

Just be sensible: Tan up gently and keep it there. Naturally dark-skinned people have to work harder. We know that African Americans suffer more from vitamin D starvation compared to Caucasians.[20]

Along with not getting enough sunshine, most people today do not get enough sun*light:* Contrary to what we believed, foragers received maximum sunlight in the morning, with a peak at 9 a.m.[21] From that time on, the foragers sought the shade if possible. The researchers opine that this phenomenon could explain why light in the morning works best for many ailments, notably depression. It is also vital for keeping the body clock synchronized. It tunes up the immune system, suppresses oxidative stress, and improves sleep quality at night.

Our ancient ancestors slept out of doors and woke up to the bright tropical morning sunlight. So, over the eons, did our bodies come to rely on it being there? "Yes," says a recent study. It finds that the timing, intensity, and duration of light exposure we get regulates how fat we get.[22] People who had good light exposure in the morning were significantly trimmer than those who did not—even though they ate the same number of calories! Light is essential to synchronize the body clock with daily bio-rhythms, which in turn regulate energy balance.

Today, say the researchers, most people do not get enough light in the morning since they work indoors. Even an overcast day is enough, whereas artificial lighting is too low to trigger the benefits.

It has long been known that people who desynchronize the body clock—e.g., by regularly working night shifts or crossing time zones (jet lag)—struggle more with obesity, diabetes, and other conditions.

The message is to get more natural light between 8 a.m. and 12 noon. At least twenty to thirty minutes is ideal, but the more the better.

SLEEPING PATTERNS

Our ancient ancestors (and forager tribes like the San) slept according to the rhythms of light and dark. In the tropics, whatever the season, dusk comes around 6 p.m. and dawn around 6 a.m. For a few hours after dusk, the San huddle around the campfire talking quietly and doing tasks by the firelight. Sleep would come around 9:30 p.m. and they would wake up with the sun.

The creatures from whom we are descended, *Homo erectus*, discovered fire at least 1 million years ago. We can imagine the nights with strange, unknown rustlings in the dark; the campfire must have been a great comfort. We all feel, even today, the fascination of a fire: Gazing reflectively into the flames is a pleasure deeply anchored in our psyches. Campfires constitute a flickering island of reassurance going back to the beginning of human existence. This is our naturally adapted prelude to sleep.

Up until the beginning of the twentieth century, populations, even in the West, did not have the luxury of much light after dark. They just had flickering whale-oil lamps and beef-fat candles; people still followed ancient ancestral sleep rhythms. Since 1900, light at night gradually became more common, first with gas lighting, then with electric light, and finally with television and electronic devices. The net result is that we do not prepare our brains for sleep in the way nature envisaged. Today, the average American sleeps two hours fewer than in the 1960s.[23] He or she certainly sleeps less—and less well—than the ideal for which our naturally adapted sleeping pattern has programmed us. Some of the consequences are predictable:

- Loss of concentration.[24]
- Lowered resistance to stress.[25]
- Depressed immune system.[25]
- Increased risk of cancer.[26]
- Increased risk of diabetes.[27]

- Increased risk of obesity.[28]
- Reduced appetite-suppressing hormones, such as leptin.[28]
- Increased hunger-inducing hormones, such as ghrelin—the less we sleep, the more we overeat![28]

Now researchers have found yet another reason for sleep. It is the time when the brain has a detox.[29] The brain and spinal cord have a circulatory system (similar to the lymphatic system) called the *glymphatic* system. During sleep, the sluices (channels) open up and the brain gets a good rinse with cerebrospinal fluid. Notably, it flushes out a toxic compound involved in Alzheimer's called beta-amyloid.

Down through the eons, humans went to sleep in mid-evening and woke with the cold—an hour before sunrise. They slept an average of seven to eight hours and often had a siesta in the heat of the day. This pattern is the ideal for us too!

PHYSICAL ACTIVITY

Earlier, we saw how the women in forager societies walked some 3 to 4 miles a day, carrying loads and with the ever-present toddler on their backs. The men walked and ran farther, but not necessarily every day. So if this were the physical activity for eons, we can be sure our bodies came to depend on it! Without it, things start to go wrong. Let me give you a few instances that you might not have thought of:

• Our heart does a good job of pumping blood around the body except for one area—the lower leg. Bedridden people and couch potatoes have circulation problems there. Why? Because the body didn't have to concern itself—it could rely on us walking around, and that action acts as a secondary pump to provide the necessary circulation in the lower leg.

• We have another circulation system—the lymphatic system—and it doesn't have a pump at all! All down the eons, it could rely on us walking around, moving our muscles to keep the circulation going. Without it, things go wrong. Immune system cells are not delivered to where they fight cancers and infections, toxic waste is not carried away, many other vital functions are lost, and the system stagnates.

• Astronauts lose 4 percent of bone mass per month when in space, no matter how many calcium pills they swallow![30] Our bone-building cells expect to receive the signaling from load-bearing physical activity to function properly. Without it, bones don't get remodeled properly, and this is a factor in osteoporosis.

• Physical activity is also one of the processes which involve hormonal responses. The body's biochemical equilibrium is designed on the assumption that it will always be there. If not, things start to go wrong. Mood and glucose control are just a couple of examples. Without the physical activity, you are more likely to be depressed, get dementia, and develop diabetes.

But the physical activity doesn't have to be intense and you don't have to be an Olympic athlete. For example, regular golfers, on average, live five years longer than non-golfers. And what do you know? They walk several miles a day, they get plenty of sunshine, and it is no coincidence that a golf course looks like an English country park, proxy for our savanna homeland.

You don't necessarily have to go out and exercise. Until fifty years ago, before all the labor-saving devices, people got enough physical activity just living their daily lives. Even a housewife today with all her running around supermarkets gets quite close. Try parking the car 100 yards from the supermarket entrance and carrying your bags instead of using a trolley.

Indeed, it is as important to avoid sitting for too long as it is to exercise. For example, think about using a standing desk when working at the computer.

STRESS

This is the fifth and final aspect of Paleolithic lifestyle that I treat in this work.

Stress always served a useful role in forager times—that is, when it is a manageable response. However, abnormal stress levels triggered in abnormal amounts is a major factor in many modern diseases. The approach of a lion, for example, must have given rise to the same emotions as a registered letter from the IRS would give us today. It also triggered another immediate categorical response: Flight.

The mismatch between our savanna-bred *mentality* and our way of life today triggers stresses several times a day that were only designed to be invoked a few times a year.

Modern living stretches and amputates us into behaviors that cut across our natures, leading to unnatural stress. We turn it on for months on end, worrying about mortgages, relationships, and promotions. We have the tyranny of the clock and the timetable. Many of us are living like neurotic caged animals.

However, unlike with the diets and foods discussed elsewhere in this guide, it is not possible to give you prescriptions. All we can do is *heighten your awareness*. Study your own circumstances in the light of this new knowledge. The examples I give in the section "Environment" (see page 26) will allow you to see how you can better realign the organization of your life so that it is more in harmony with your human psyche.

This is a vast topic and we look at just a few themes in this work. In Chapter 3, I will discuss how our modern eating patterns have come to be such a mismatch from those of the foraging societies of our ancient ancestors.

3.

How Did It Go Wrong?

As you have read, our foraging ancestors had certain feeding, sleeping, physical activity, and working patterns that they adhered to. In the Western world today, we no longer follow any of these patterns, and as a result we are afflicted with conditions (such as obesity, heart disease, and diabetes) that were unknown to our ancestors. So when—and how—did it all go wrong?

As we saw, 60,000 years ago, our ancestors were multiplying fast. They moved out of Africa and, by 12,000 years ago, they had occupied every corner of the globe. But they still needed 200 square miles per forager band, so they were fighting each other for living space.

Then 11,000 years ago, a group of people discovered a solution: They took control of their food supply. Instead of taking their chances, they made sure that most of what was growing in their area was edible. So instead of living on 200 square miles, they could live on 2 square miles. People started to farm.

But there were two difficulties with this. First of all, they reduced right down the *variety* of plant foods from over 100 species to just three or four. This is important because, as we saw in Chapter 1, humans are primarily fruit-salad-plant eaters. Our bodies, our digestive systems and, above all, our biochemistries rely on an intake of a vast variety of nutrients, micronutrients, minerals, and vitamins. By focusing on just three or four staples, those first farmers suffered from all kinds of micronutrient deficiencies. And the same goes for us today, too!

Second, these first farmers planted not what they were used to eating, but what it was *possible* to cultivate, harvest, and store through the winter months. And so it was, for the first time in the history of the human race, people started to eat bird seed! Alright, that is being provocative, but it's important to make the point sink home: Bird seed is just what *cereals* are—and the first cereals were *wheat* and *barley*. They were followed by rice, oats, rye, and corn (maize).

In this chapter, I will discuss the consequences of eating farmed, manufactured, and processed foods. These foods include cereals (grains), potatoes, sugar, beans (legumes), hydrogenated oils, and dairy. It may seem overwhelming to strictly limit or eliminate all of these food groups from your diet, but in the Owner's Manual (see page 53), I will present a guide that will help you implement the Paleo style of eating into your daily life.

THE PROBLEM WITH CEREALS

First, let's be clear: When we talk of cereals (or grains) we also mean everything we make from them—bread, pastries, pasta, breakfast cereals, cakes, muffins, popcorn, and so forth. So why are these foods so bad for us, and what is wrong with cereals?

Starch

First of all, cereals and grains are *starchy*. And starch is just another form of sugar—a slice of toast actually hits the bloodstream faster than a teaspoon of sugar.[1] So right here, we are careering off on that injurious blood sugar and insulin switchback that I discussed in Chapter 2.

Micronutrient Poor

Do you get a warm feeling when you see that your breakfast cereal is "fortified" with a list of vitamins and minerals? How good of the manufacturers! In truth, even the government knows that cereals are rubbish food. The government requires the food processors to do most of this "enrichment" because without this interference, grains are, quite naturally, *poor in micronutrients*. By eating grains, we are starving our bodies of the tens of thousands of micronutrients that our bodies need—the ones which quench inflammation and feed the immune system.

Anti-nutrients

All plants secrete chemicals to protect themselves from insects, bacteria, viruses, and funguses. Creatures, like us, who evolved to eat certain types of plants (corresponding to our fruits, salads, and vegetables), have bodies which know how to handle their chemicals. In a way, these chemicals are plant poisons—but not poisons to us.

That works fine in a state of nature. But now, the farmers are making us eat a new food group—grasses (grains) which contain plant poisons that our bodies have not met before and do not know how to handle. For us, these plant poisons are indeed poisonous, working silently in the background to undermine our health.

Gluten (a glue-like protein found in grains) is an obvious example, but others are lectins, alpha-amylase inhibitors, and many more. They do things like:

- Make our colons more porous. This is sometimes called "leaky colon" or "leaky gut." The gut wall, which is as thin as tissue paper, becomes abnormally porous and so allows bacteria, funguses, food particles, allergens, antigens, and other harmful molecules to pass through and into the blood and lymph systems, where they create mischief and undermine general health.[2]

- Disrupt red blood cells.[3]

- Depress human growth hormone (and so undermine cell renewal).[4]

- Neutralize pancreatic hormones (driving it to step up production to the point of failure).[5]

- Disrupt DNA maintenance, allowing mutations to flourish.[6]

Not Alkalizing

Finally, grains are not alkalizing. They are mildly acidic, so by eating breads, pastas, and so forth, we are shouldering aside the types of plant foods that *are* alkalizing.

As we saw in the section "It Helps to Know What We Are Not" on page 18, humans are not granivores. Grains are for the birds!

POTATO

Now, we come to a tuber which Chaucer had never heard of and which Shakespeare only knew as pig-fattening food. Yet, just in the last 200 years, the potato has come to dominate our diet. But the potato suffers the same drawbacks as grains:

- It is starchy and so glycemic and insulinemic.[7]

- It is empty of micronutrients.[8]

- It can have sickening levels of plant poisons (also called glycoalkaloids).[9]

- It is not alkalizing.[10]

Potato consumption is directly linked to allergies, bowel disorders, confusion, and depression. Every year, dozens of people are hospitalized with potato poisoning, and many more cases go undiagnosed. These problems are directly linked to the anti-nutrients in the potato that our bodies can't cope with.

SUGAR

Unlike potatoes and processed grains, sugar was not unknown to our ancestors—but it was rare. There was not much sweetness in foragers' lives, apart from their loved ones! Just about the only source of sugar was honey. Indeed, foragers prized it highly and went to a lot of trouble to get it. However, they did have help in the form of the honeyguide bird. This extraordinary bird called to a forager and guided him to a bees' nest. The forager climbed the tree, chopped open the hole, smoked the bees out, reached in, and—in spite of the stings—pulled out handfuls of honeycomb. It was partly filled with honey and partly with bee larvae. Foragers took a mouthful and, after sucking out the edible parts (larvae and all), spit out the wax.[11]

In exchange, the honeyguide got the remaining honeycomb in the nest. This is a wonderful example of two species working together for mutual benefit. For this behavior to become hardwired into a bird's brain, it must have been going on for eons.

This means that, even in Paleolithic times, honey must have been important to both forager and honeyguide—yet, this aspect is routinely glossed over in reconstructing the Paleo diet. But now the evidence points to the fact that honey provided a significant proportion of calories to our Paleo forebears.[12,13]

For large parts of more recent human history, honey was a rare commodity. But then came sugar—and sugar is just honey in another form. The sugarcane, and its sweet sap, was known in ancient Asia. However, it had little impact until commercial interests, just in the last 200 years, learned how to refine its sap into sugar on an industrial scale and spread their sugarcane plantations into all propitious areas of the tropical world.

Since that time in the eighteenth century, consumption rocketed from some 4 lbs per head per year to the point where Americans today are consuming some 140 lbs/head/year.[14] That's a massive 3,500 percent increase in the consumption of this highly metabolically active substance. Intake has gone from a condiment quantity—which the body joyfully accepts and handles perfectly well—to one that creates the havoc with our biochemistry we reviewed on page 24.

We can say that honey—or less ideally, sugar—has a place in Paleo nutrition, but it should be strictly limited. That's the challenge. Processed, manufactured, and other fake foods are riddled with hidden sugar (or its evil twin, high fructose corn syrup): Breakfast cereals, muffins, pasta sauces, dressings, smoothies, desserts (of course), sweets, canned fruits, and so forth. Even bread is adulterated with it. That is to say nothing about fruit juices, sodas, and colas—they take you over the limit in one go.

So the strategy has to be this: Do everything you can to strip processed foods from the diet. Only when you are eating entirely generic food in its original state (and that you are not getting *any* hidden sugars at all) can you permit yourself to add back in a few teaspoons of honey a day—just like your ancestral forager!

THE TROUBLE WITH BEANS

Let's now back up in time to those ingenious first farmers. Along with grains (cereals), they also got us eating yet another new food group: *Legumes* (pulses). That is, they grew *beans* and *lentils*.

Many of us have probably wondered if we are naturally adapted to eating beans, considering that they give us gas—and the gases are greenhouse gases like methane, hydrogen, and carbon dioxide. So by eating beans, we are contributing to global warming! Although that is a stretch, it is a humorous way of making a point: There is a whole range of new foodstuffs that have entered our diet over the last 2,000 generations. We think of them as normal, traditional human foods, but they are not. We have discovered only in the last few years that many of these new foods are making us sick in ways that no one suspected.

The beans story highlights a point: Our bodies don't know how to handle beans—and it matters. In particular, they contain anti-nutrients similar to grains (see page 35).[15] Some of the anti-nutrients are so potent that packets of dry beans warn to cook them thoroughly for at least ten minutes. This weakens the poisons sufficiently enough not to cause obvious harm, but underneath, they are still silently doing their mischief.

Until recently, beans were not a major constituent of the Western diet (only about 4 lbs per person per year were consumed in the U.S.) and we could safely ignore them. No longer. Just in the last twenty-five years, one bean has become all-pervasive: The *soy* bean. It is in everything: Bread, cookies, and all kinds of processed foods. Some people eat it directly as tofu, in yogurt, and as soy protein.

As a bean, soy is tarred with the same brush. It has its share of plant poisons (such as lectins, genistein, daidzein, trypsin inhibitors, allergens, and phytoe-strogens). The wonders of marketing have turned these drawbacks into advantages: Women are sold soy as a remedy for conditions such as hot flashes and PMS. It is even sold as having anti-cancer properties, when in fact it increases the risk of uterine cancer,[16] breast cancer,[17] and pancreatic cancer. Soy's anti-nutrients genistein and daidzein attack thyroid function,[18] which can lead to goiter and, in extreme cases, thyroid cancer.

Soy gives you brain atrophy: The more people eat soy bean curds (tofu), for example, the more likely they are to have senile dementia in later life. Dr. Lon White, a researcher on aging, studied Japanese Americans in Hawaii and found that consumption of only two portions of tofu a week raises the chances of getting dementia by 50 percent, compared with consumption of no tofu at all.[19] Soybeans contain a lectin that undermines the immune system by messing with the membrane of its cells, called "lymphocytes."[20]

Finally, soy is a well-known allergen. Those of you who frequent the "allergy-free" shelves of the supermarket will know this. Indeed, over sixteen allergens have been identified in soy, of which at least three are considered "severe."[21]

In conclusion, legumes (including soy) are not human food and they contribute to sickness, usually in sneaky, subtle ways that are not immediately obvious to us.

TIME FOR AN OIL CHANGE?

When we think of our savanna homeland, there was not much fat around. Most animals had little body fat (around 4 percent) and there were no bottles of peanut oil hanging from the trees! Even so, humans have a strong yen for fatty foods and our forager ancestors sought it out avidly. They found it chiefly in bone marrow, brains, and tree nuts like the mongongo and baobab. Added up, fat provided some 25 percent of calories—well below the average for modern Americans (33 percent[22]) but more than traditional Japanese (10 percent).

The fat levels are important, but much more importantly, they had a particular fatty acid *profile:* That is, the fats were of a specific kind and were present in particular ratios to each other.

To keep it simple, I will focus just on two fatty acids that were always present in such a way that our bodies never had to learn to make them. They are *essential* and without them we sicken and die. Because of this, we call them *essential fatty acids.*

The Power of Essential Fatty Acids

You have probably heard of two fatty acids called *omega-3* and *omega-6.* Even small amounts of these two essential fatty acids have powerful effects on the body—much like hormones do. And they operate in opposing ways: What one does, the other undoes. For example, one increases blood clotting, the other decreases it; one increases blood pressure, the other decreases blood pressure—and so on. This is a summary:

OMEGA-3	CONDITIONS	OMEGA-6
Reduces	Allergies (histamines)	Increases
Reduces	Alzheimer's, dementia	Increases
Reduces	Artery hardening	Increases
Reduces	Asthma (vasoconstriction)	Increases
Increases	Bone building	Reduces
Reduces	Blood clotting (thromboses)	Increases
Reduces	Blood pressure	Increases
Reduces	Cancer	Increases
Reduces	Cholesterol	Increases
Reduces	Inflammation	Increases
Reduces	Insulin levels	Increases
Reduces	Pain sensitivity	Increases

Both of these fatty acids are essential for survival; omega-3 and omega-6 need to be present in roughly equal amounts. As a rule of thumb, the body can cope with imbalances of up to 3 to 1. This was precisely the case under savanna life: The see-saw was just gently oscillating up and down with the hazards of food intake.

What we have done today is drastically *un*balance this see-saw: The omega-6 fatty acid totally dominates the conversion pathway. On average, Americans are eating *thirty times* as much omega-6 as omega-3![23] It firmly fastens the see-saw down at one end, as shown in Figure 3.1 below.

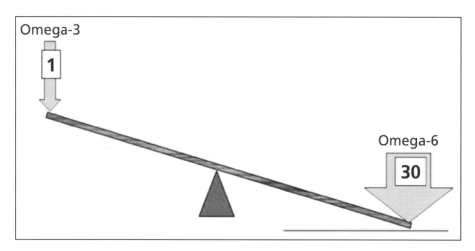

Figure 3.1. Modern imbalance of the omega-3 to omega-6 ratio.

How has this happened? Today, these are the major sources of omega-6 and omega-3 oils in the Western diet:

OMEGA-6	OMEGA-3
• Sunflower oil	• Canola/rapeseed oil
• Corn/maize oil	• Omega-3 rich eggs
• Peanut oil	• Flax oil, borage oil, hempseed oil
• Safflower oil	• Oily fish: salmon, sardines, herring, mackerel, trout, etc.

Just in my lifetime, omega-6 oils have come to dominate the diet. "Well," you may say, "They are *good,* aren't they—they are vegetable oils!" However, they are not good in excess—and their domination happened because in the 1960s, we became anxious about the horrors of saturated fat and were persuaded to use vegetable oil instead of pork lard and beef dripping.

The shift in consumption was meteoric: Consumption of omega-6 vegetable oils rocketed from 12 lbs per head per year in 1965 to 50 lbs per head per year today—that's a 400 percent increase![24] In parallel, consumption of fish declined and food manufacturers stripped omega-3 oil out of their products—why?

Because it goes rancid easily and so has a short shelf life, equaling a lower monetary profit for food manufacturers.

We only need about one gram each of omega-6 and omega-3 oils. We need to strip out the omega-6 oils to the point where we are only consuming a couple of grams a day *at most*, and we need to make sure we get *at least* one gram a day of omega-3 oils. Eating oily fish every day will help you boost your intake of omega-3.

Other Fats and Oils

Up until now, we have focused on *essential* fats or oils. Omega-3 and omega-6 oils are polyunsaturated fats. But what about monounsaturated fat, like olive oil? What about saturated fats, hydrogenated fats, and trans fats? This section will discuss each of these types of fat.

Monounsaturated Fats

Monounsaturated fats were quite common in our ancestral environment, particularly in the marrow of bones and many nuts. Our bodies know how to handle them in a healthy way. Health benefits of monounsaturated fats include lowering cholesterol levels, reducing the risk of heart disease and stroke, and enhancing cell building and the immune system. Today, our most common source is olive oil. Avocado is another good source.

Saturated Fat of Animal Origin

Saturated fats from animal products have received a bad rap since the 1960s, when a link was found with hardening of the arteries and cardiovascular disease. This observation applied particularly to the fat from "red meat" farm animals (beef, pork, and lamb) and from dairy fats (butter and cream). Indeed, the types of fatty acid found in these foods, *palmitic* and *myristic,* are ones that were rare in our ancestral diets. Large amounts overwhelm our bodies' ability to deal with them, leading to high triglycerides, high cholesterol, and increased risk of cardiovascular disease.[25] The amount and type of fat found in animal products largely depends on how the animals are raised and fed (see inset "It Matters How We Feed Our Animals" on page 42).

Saturated Fats of Plant Origin

Certain saturated fats derived from plants, like coconut oil and cocoa butter, have become a fetish consumption by some health mavens. Actually, none of these fats was common in our savanna environment but, by a quirk of triglyceride biochemistry, their *palmitic* and *myristic* acids (the harmful fatty acids found in saturated fats) are not readily bioavailable. This means they are not readily taken in by the body. As a result, they do not have the devastating effect on our biochemistry that those fats of animal origin do. We see absolutely no

It Matters How We Feed Our Animals

As long ago as 1968, Dr. Michael Crawford (then of the London Zoo) made groundbreaking research on the body fat in African animals.[26] He discovered that the kinds of body fats present changed vastly according to what the animals fed on:

- Wild buffalo living in their natural woodland habitat feed on low-lying bushes. Their body fat had a high percentage (30 percent) of the two "good" polyunsaturated fats. And their omega-6 level was within the good ratio of 3:1 with omega-3.

- Wild buffalo living in parkland (grassland with only occasional bushes and trees) had much poorer percentages (8 percent) of polyunsaturated fat.

- African grass-fed farm cattle had only 2 percent polyunsaturated fat.

- Other studies show that the more corn a cow is fed, the worse is its omega-3 intake.[27]

- Moreover, wild giraffes (which feed off treetops) had 39 percent polyunsaturated fat, while zoo giraffes (which feed on hay) had only 4 percent.

These differences were found in humans, too: American mothers had only 8 percent polyunsaturated fat in their breast milk, while the breast milk of Japanese women contained 25 percent.

Crawford made the point that, whether it is Africa or Europe, grassland is not the countryside's natural state; on the contrary, bushes and trees make up our natural landscape. Crawford went on to suggest that humans, in creating unnatural habitats for farm animals, are upsetting the various body-fat balances. He proposed that this will have harmful consequences for humans who eat farmed animal products.

In another 1968 study, Crawford made the connection between heart disease and the conventional, but unnatural, way we feed farm animals.[28]

reason to consume these plant-derived saturated fats but, if you do, your body will probably not suffer from them.

Hydrogenated and Trans Fats

There is nothing good to say about hydrogenated fats or trans fats. These artificial horrors were invented as a way to convert vegetable oils into solid fat. In so doing, manufacturers created a Darth Vader for our arteries. Quite rightly, health authorities demonize them and some jurisdictions ban them outright.

Oil Change Summary

The chart below lists the most commonly consumed oils. Each oil is categorized as "favorable" (the first choice you should pick), "conforming" (safe choices that are good alternatives to the "favorable" oils), "tolerated" (acceptable choices, but should only be used if necessary), or "avoid."

FAVORABLE	CONFORMING	TOLERATED	AVOID
Canola/rapeseed oil	Olive oil	Palm oil	Sunflower oil
Oily fish	Walnut oil	Coconut oil	Safflower oil
Omega-3 eggs	Soybean oil	Cocoa butter	Corn oil
Flax oil			Peanut oil
Hempseed oil			Butter, cream
Borage oil			Animal fats, lard, dripping
			Hydrogenated/trans fat

DAIRY

About 5,000 years ago, a tribe of cow and sheep herders on the steppes in what is now Ukraine developed the odd idea of consuming the secretions from the mammary glands of their lactating animals—a humorous way of saying that they consumed cow's milk and sheep's milk. These people migrated northwest and became the Slavs, Germans, Anglo-Saxons, and Scandinavians.

By 2,000 years ago, they had made milk and its products into a staple—they invented dairy farming as a major industry. From about the year 1600 these peoples migrated to North America, Australia, and New Zealand, carrying their idea of dairy consumption with them.

But we forget that they only represent 20 percent of the world's population. The remaining 80 percent—Asians, Africans, Latin Americans, etc.—not only think that milk consumption is bizarre and grotesque, it makes them sick!

What about our template, the hunter-gatherer? Correct, Bushmen were not creeping around under female antelopes, suckling their teats! So let us examine this curious practice in this way: The milk of a species is for the young of *that* species. For example, cow's milk is designed to be food for young cows—not young humans. As we saw in the "What We Are Not" section on page 18, we simply don't have the digestive enzymes, the biochemistry, or the biology for milk consumption past the age of about three years old.

I like to put it like this: A newborn mammal is really an unfinished fetus— it is at an intermediate stage, like a chrysalis before it becomes a butterfly. A mother's milk is basically fetus-finishing food. So, by consuming milk—to put it provocatively—we are consuming fetus food. And by drinking cow's milk we are, to put it provocatively again, consuming a fluid that is designed to build small brains and big horns! Is that what we want for ourselves and our families?

I've poked some fun at the practice of consuming dairy and its products, but we do know that there are real problems, as I discuss in the following sections.

Bad Dairy Fats

When I was a kid, we used to think that the cream at the top of the milk bottle was the best part. But in the 1960s, the scientists started warning that this cream is an unhealthy saturated fat (the dreaded myristic and palmitic acids of animal origin), and we are better off using skimmed milk. Skim milk is not really any better, however, as it still contains lactose and milk proteins.

Lactose—A Bad Allergen

More recently, we have become aware of another drawback—lactose. This is the naturally occurring sugar in milk that requires the special enzyme *lactase* to digest it.

As we saw earlier with the San Bushmen in "What Was Their Health Like?" (see page 16), in a state of nature, we stop making lactose as we grow up. Many people of northwest European extraction (i.e., descendants of the first dairy farmers) continue to produce lactase well into adulthood, but even their production usually tapers off in middle age.

These days, we can buy milk that has had both the fat and the lactose removed. You might ask, "Then why are we bothering with this stuff?" But the mischief hasn't finished: There is still the problem of the milk proteins.

Bad Dairy Proteins

Milk is one of the top eight allergens recognized by the U.S. Federal Government. This means that, by law, any food products containing milk must be properly labeled. Often, what gives people an allergic reaction to milk is the milk proteins. One of the major proteins in dairy is *casein*. A second is *lactalbumin* (found in the whey). Both of these are allergenic. Non-human milk (e.g., cow's milk) also contains a protein unknown to human biology: *Beta-lactoglobulin*. This, too, is allergenic.

Casein also raises levels of IGF-1—an *insulin-like growth factor* implicated in inflammation and cancer.[29]

The Unknown Unknowns

Finally, let us not forget that cow's milk is designed to turn a newborn calf into a mature cow as quickly as possible. So it quite naturally contains a variety of highly active compounds: Growth factors, hormones, enzymes, antibodies, bacteria, and immune stimulants. But these are meant for baby cows—what effect do they have on grown-up humans? We don't know—we still don't even know what many of these compounds are or what they do, exactly.

Bone Health and the Calcium Myth

Now to dispel a myth. I am frequently asked: If you don't eat dairy, where do you get your calcium? I respond by asking a question of my own. How do cows build bones? By eating grass! But I find that the American philosopher Henry Thoreau, in his book *Walden*, put it more elegantly in 1854: "One farmer says to me, 'You cannot live on vegetable food solely, for it furnishes nothing to make bones with'...walking all the while behind his oxen, which, with vegetable-made bones, jerk him and his plow along..."

The typical dietetic mantra is that we only have to swill down calcium by the bucketful to avoid osteoporosis. There cannot be more humbug spoken about bone health. We see gorillas, oxen, and elephants building massive bones just out of vegetation. No, there are other factors at work besides calcium.

Statistics on the incidence of hip fractures find that Norwegians (for example) have five times the rate of hip fractures as that of Spaniards.[30] What is it that Spaniards are doing differently?

One answer is that they do not consume dairy products as frequently. Another piece of evidence can be found in the famous Nurses Health Study, which has been running since 1976. The study published in 1997 found that those women who drank two or more glasses of milk a day were 40 percent more likely to have hip fractures than those who drank none.[31] This goes against everything you have been told!

Researchers found no signs of osteoporosis in the San Bushmen, even though they do not drink milk or swallow calcium pills.[32] The dairy-free populations of Asia and Africa, although consuming modest levels of calcium, do not suffer from bone fractures.[33] Finally, just because calcium gets into the bloodstream, it does not mean that the body uses it to build bones. On the contrary, the body is quite capable of laying down calcium just where you do not want it. For example, calcium can be placed in the arteries and heart valves (as plaque); in the kidneys (as stones); in the breasts (as nodules triggering cancers); and in the joints (as painful spurs).[34,35] All this can happen while the bones themselves are losing calcium. Clearly something is very wrong with the conventional doctrine.

The thing to understand is this: The bones are like a lattice structure, something like the Eiffel Tower, where the struts are made of calcium phosphate and the rivets are made of collagen. Conventionally, all the focus on bone health is on the calcium struts. But bone falls apart if the collagen deteriorates, too! The bones are undergoing a constant process of destruction and rebuilding. In a lifetime, our skeletons are replaced three times over.

All this bone refurbishment takes place with cells (osteoclasts) that crawl over the lattice, pulling out weak struts and its collagen attachment. They talk to bone-building cells (osteoblasts) to come and put a new strut back with a strong new collagen glue. The osteoblasts talk to the gut, saying: "Next time you see a calcium molecule coming along, allow it through the gut wall and pop it into the bloodstream so that we can pick it up." In fact, there is a myriad of little instructions going to and fro between various parts of the body to make all this happen.

And what we do with our lifestyle is interrupt these messages, or send the wrong signals. The net result is that the osteoclasts speed up and the osteoblasts slow down. A summary of the major factors is shown in the table below:

Bone Building Factors	Bone Dismantling Factors
Micronutrient rich diet	Dairy products
Good gut microbe signaling	Bad gut microbe signaling
Good sunshine exposure	Gluten (wheat, rye, and barley products)
Brain serotonin signaling	Acid diet
Physical activity	High phosphorus (e.g., cola) diet
Sex hormone functionality	High insulin levels (high glycemic diet)
Constructive kidney signaling	High salt intake
	Omega-6 oils
	Disruptive kidney signaling

Quite why the consumption of dairy undermines bone health is not clear. The main reason seems to be that it provokes *inflammation*—which in turn destroys bone. Dairy also adds to the acidic load of a diet, which, as we saw in Chapter 1, also weakens bone.

When all is said and done, we do know that dairy and its products are factors in a range of illnesses:[31,36,37,38,39,40,41]

- Cancers
- Heart disease
- Osteoporosis
- Cholesterol
- Allergies
- Migraine
- Irritable bowel, colitis
- ADHD
- Arthritis

So far in our examination of dairy products, we have focused on milk. But what about other dairy products, like cheese and yogurt?

Cheese

Cheese is perhaps the "least bad" of the dairy products. Its lactose mostly disappears in the fermentation process and its fats, seemingly, are poorly absorbed by the body.[42] So you could occasionally treat yourself to a nice ripe Stilton or camembert with a glass of red wine.

Yogurt

I would reserve a special circle of Hell for this pesky product. Most of us in the industrial West had never heard of it until, in the 1980s, the magic of marketing made it obligatory to consume by the trusting, but duped, health-conscious. It has all the drawbacks of milk itself and, as we have seen on page 22, it can be highly insulinemic to boot.[43] Its boasted probiotic property—a cargo of "good" gut bacteria—is fool's gold. It is unlikely that any bacteria from yogurt make it through the stomach's acid bath to get to the colon and, even if they did, as we saw in "Our Living Gut" on page 23, it is futile and counterproductive to inject just one or two species into a wildly chaotic menagerie of bacterial agents. Avoid!

THE PALEO FORMULA

Now that we have cleared out all the non-human foods, let us survey what is left. In my view, it is most conveniently presented as a food pyramid (see Figure 3.2 below)—just like the authorities used to do before they kept changing their ideas about what to recommend.

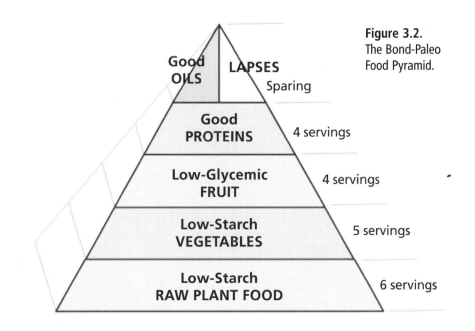

Figure 3.2.
The Bond-Paleo Food Pyramid.

As an aside, please note that in this segment we will summarize just the basic principles. For a full schedule of Paleo-conforming foodstuffs, see the Owner's Manual on page 53.

Let us start at the bottom layer and work our way up. At the bottom (the largest part of the pyramid, indicating those foods we should be consuming the most), we do not have all the breads, starches, pastas, and breakfast cereals that the authorities want us to consume. Instead, we have *low-starch raw plant food*. It is quite easy really to achieve six servings by eating one big salad every day with all the usual ingredients we think of as salad vegetables: Tomatoes, lettuce, radish, cucumber, mushrooms, onions, and so forth.

Next up are the *low-starch vegetables* (five servings). These are the usual items we call vegetables, such as green beans, broccoli, and kale—with the exception of potato, of course. We should also go easy on sweet potato, carrots, and peas, which are starchy-sugary and moderately glycemic.

Low-glycemic fruits are on the third layer (four servings). Fruits in our ancestral homeland were much less sugary and less watery than most of the fruits we have today. However, most berries (raspberries, blueberries, redcurrants, strawberries, etc.) are low-glycemic; grapefruit, apples, bananas, and many other fruits are also okay. But we have to go easy on sweet, sugary fruits like pineapple, mango, and melons.

On the next layer are *good proteins* (four servings). Omega-3 rich/fortified eggs are fine—but best of all, if you can get them, are farmyard eggs from hens that have been scratching around eating insects, worms, seeds, and greenery (like purslane). All seafood is good, particularly the oily fish. Most poultry is conforming, particularly duck and goose and even turkey. If you can get wild game like pheasant and grouse, that is good. However, do avoid battery chickens (chickens raised in tiny, individual cages)—their fatty acid profile is terrible. And, if you can get them, the exotic meats like venison, crocodile, ostrich, and caribou are good too.

In fact, most animal matter is okay, so long as it isn't beef, lamb, or especially, pork. Our bodies simply can't handle their fatty acid profiles, with the grievous consequences to our health that we all know about. All tree nuts are acceptable sources of good protein, as well as products made from them (for examples, see the recipes for Paleo breads, muffins, and cakes in the companion cookbook *Paleo Harvest*).

Good oils share the top of the pyramid, and should be eaten sparingly to reap their health benefits. Refer to the fats I itemize in "Time for an Oil Change" (see page 38). These include oily fish and canola (rapeseed) oil.

Lapses are at the top of the pyramid as well. These are the unhealthy foods in which we "indulge" from time to time. Reserve these for special occasions like your birthday or a wedding anniversary. And don't become habituated to them!

WHAT ABOUT DRINKING?

Typically, foragers lived in an area which had lakes and streams. They would camp a few hundred yards away so as to not scare the game. Were they constantly guzzling lake water? No—they got a high percentage of fluid from the foods they ate. Indeed, San Bushmen (who do live in very marginal areas) have been observed to go without free water for 280 days!

We are certainly not recommending that you try to do that. However, in total contrast, today we are bombarded with scare messages claiming that we are in all mortal danger of dehydration.

However, as Dr. Heinz Valtin (a kidney expert with the department of physiology at Dartmouth Medical School) said, it's "difficult to believe that evolution left us with a chronic water deficit that needs to be compensated by forcing a high fluid intake."[44]

In this context, it is worth mentioning that most people today are eating foodstuffs that are low in water, and so they feel thirsty more frequently. Once you start eating Paleo, with its water-rich vegetation, you will find that you will need to drink less.

Thirst Doesn't Mean Dehydration

It is often claimed that by the time people feel thirsty, they are already dehydrated. On the contrary, thirst begins when the blood has become less dilute by under 2 percent, whereas dehydration begins when the blood has become less dilute by at least 5 percent. When we were kids and were thirsty, we just ran up to a tap and gulped from it. Now the authorities are backing this principle.[45] Let thirst be your guide—you do not *have* to drink water if you are not thirsty. (See "The 8x8 Myth" below.)

It actually is possible to have *too much* water. Many ordinary folk have died of water intoxication, fondly believing the mantra, "The more water, the better."

The 8x8 Myth

Where did the 8x8 myth (the idea that we must drink at least eight 8-ounce cups of water a day) come from? Nobody knows! The nearest clue we have is that back in the 1940s, the Food and Nutrition Board opined that daily fluid intake should be around 64 fluid ounces (8 x 8-ounce cups). But this recommendation came with the proviso that most of the fluids would come from food. Then, with the magic of modern marketing in the 1980s, we were persuaded to buy water from a bottle and glug from it at every opportunity. Many of the arguments are manipulative and utterly spurious: For example, that drinking all this water helps to lose weight, or that it "detoxifies the body."

With regard to athletes, Dr. Deborah Cohen (investigations editor of the *British Medical Journal*) observed that no marathon runner has suffered from dehydration, whereas some sixteen marathon runners have died from over-hydration (water intoxication) and 1,600 were made critically ill. She found that sports drink companies sponsor scientists dedicated to promoting hydration.[46] Their greatest success was to undermine the idea that the body has a perfectly good mechanism for detecting dehydration—thirst. And so they have spread false alarms about the "dangers" of dehydration.

Water and What Else?

While our forager forebears had no way of boiling water or making infusions, in this regard we agree with the USDA's advice: Suitable fluids can include tea, herbal tea, and coffee in moderation. In the great scheme of things, caffeine is not a huge issue, but it is wise to go easy on it, since it does interfere with blood sugar metabolism and can irritate many other metabolic functions. I discuss this further in the Owner's Manual (see page 80).

Other fluids need to pass the usual tests—in particular, do they contain sugars or high fructose corn syrup (HFCS)? Are they glycemic? (It is usually so with fruit juices.) Do they contain much salt? And so on.

CONCLUSION

This chapter has highlighted the stark difference between what our ancestors ate and what we eat today. We have discussed how these changes have been adopted as the "Western diet" and spread worldwide over the centuries. Starting with the agricultural movement, we have ceased to seek out and eat what nature provides us and instead *create* our food. This is problematic because substances for which our digestive systems are not designed—preservatives, sugars, salt, animal milks, and so forth—are pedaled and fed to us as if they are necessary for our survival. They are not.

The next chapter contains the Owner's Manual. Consider this your guide to your digestive system. It details what you need to keep your body up and running, and what you must eliminate to prevent slowdown and illness. Do not fear going hungry—as you will find, there is a bounty of foods that we consider to be safe and delicious to eat.

PART II

Eating the Paleo Way

4.

The Owner's Manual

In Part I of this book, we painted a picture of our naturally adapted lifestyle. We saw how our ancient environment conditioned our bodies—and our very natures—for life on the savannas of East Africa. We called this lifestyle the "Savanna Model" and outlined how our ancient ancestors fed themselves for thousands of generations. This outline gives us the key to how we should be feeding ourselves today.

It's as if our bodies are incredibly complex machines for which we have lost the operating instructions, or the "Owner's Manual" as we call it here. Visualize the Owner's Manual as an ancient parchment that generations of scribes have overwritten many times. By carefully clearing away the more recent layers, we can rediscover the original scripture.

We have reviewed how the naturally adapted feeding pattern changed dramatically with the farming revolution 11,000 years ago. Governments intervene to regulate our food supply with the laudable intention of keeping it "fit" for "human consumption," but they've only had partial success. Governments also took it upon themselves to advise us how and what to eat, but much of this advice is flawed. In what follows, I redefine the conventional food groups to fit with the Paleo understanding of what is human and non-human food. In Appendix A, we look at how other populations (Eskimos, Japanese, Cretans) around the world fare with their different diets. We put the microscope on how our bodies and biochemistry operate. By seeing what works well—and what works badly—we get strong pointers to the ideal feeding patterns for the human organism.

We have now done enough to clear away all the overwritten layers of our Owner's Manual. In this part of the book, we reveal the original scripture.

There is no way that we can go back to eating the identical foods of our ancient ancestors or even those of today's San Bushmen. We are totally dependent on the modern supply chain that brings us foods from near and far, most of it farmed. The species of plant food and animal matter are quite different, too: We are not going to find caterpillars, mongongo nuts, or grewia berries in the supermarket any time soon! The way forward is to define the essential, fundamental characteristics of the Savanna Model eating pattern and then apply them in the modern world. When we put together all that we know—from foragers and foraging theory; from what goes wrong when we don't fuel our bodies correctly; from what we know about our biochemistry; from information gleaned from population studies and clinical studies—we can identify basic characteristics of the ideal human feeding pattern, for eating the way nature intended.

OWNER'S MANUAL TABLE OF CONTENTS

Here, we pull together all the arguments, evidence, and reasonings to draw up the broad outlines of the feeding pattern that is ideal for the human species. These, then, are the contents of the Owner's Manual. In the sections that follow, I will delve more into each "chapter" of the manual.

Basic Specifications

Nature designed the human feeding pattern to:

1. Be low-glycemic.

2. Be low-insulinemic.

3. Have acid-alkali ratio in balance.

4. Have a high volume of high-fiber, low-density foods.

5. Sustain a low sodium (salt) to high potassium ratio.

6. Sustain a healthy fatty acid profile.

7. Provide high micronutrient content.

8. Provide a low plant poison (anti-nutrient) level.

9. Have a low antigen content.

10. Produce hunger some of the time.

Low-Glycemic and Low-Insulinemic

We saw that the San have a diet that is rich in plant food, yet there is little in the way of starches and sugar. Their digging sticks produce plenty of tubers, but their starch content is low and difficult to extract. Blood sugar levels rise moderately and slowly. Consequently, the San insulin secretions do not have the lightning response that the bodies of us Westerners have been forced to adopt. This phenomenon is known as "insulin resistance." This is a feature that modern medicine considers to be pathological—but in reality, this is how humans are supposed to be!

Our closest cousins in the animal kingdom, the chimpanzee and the gorilla, have similar low-starch and low-sugar diets. Starches and sugars badly disturb our blood sugar control. This in turn disrupts our biochemistry, leading to numerous diseases and eventually, death. We come to the inescapable conclusion that nature designed the human frame for what we call a low-glycemic diet: That is, one that does not produce abnormal blood sugar spikes. The Western diet we have adopted, however, is the opposite—it produces high blood sugar surges. Abnormally high (and harmful) levels of insulin are the major consequence of high blood sugar levels. However, other factors too can aggravate high insulin levels, notably foods that are "high-insulinemic."

Owner's Manual: Focus on low-glycemic, low-insulinemic foods.

Acid-Alkali Balance

The San eat a diet that is roughly 75 percent plant food, which is alkali-forming, and 25 percent animal matter, which is acid-forming. They eat no grains or dairy products, which are both acid-forming. The net result is a diet that creates a neutral state in the blood between acidity and alkalinity. This is the ideal state for human biochemistry to function properly. Unfortunately, the average Western diet is strongly acidic.

Owner's Manual: Keep protein consumption modest (25 percent by weight) and keep non-starchy plant food and fruit consumption high (75 percent by weight).

High Volumes of High-Fiber, Low-Density Foods

Our evolutionary past designed our digestive systems to have high volumes of plant food passing through them. These non-starchy plant foods were, by nature, low-density: That is, they had few calories for their volume. A lettuce leaf, for example, is 95 percent water (the remaining 5 percent is a wonderful cornucopia of vital nutrients). In addition, plant food is rich in various plant fibers, the sort that our colons are designed to work with. The typical Western diet is the opposite: Energy-dense and low in fiber.

Owner's Manual: Consume high volumes of fibrous non-starchy plant foods and fruits.

Low-Sodium to High-Potassium Ratio

Salt, until very recent times, was a scarce commodity. In our ancestral homeland, it was unknown. Humans and other creatures only absorbed sodium from what was innate to the food they were eating. For example, uncooked broccoli contains, quite naturally, 27 mg of sodium per 100 g. Similarly, it contains 325 mg of potassium per 100 g. This ratio (about 1 to 12) of sodium to potassium is of fundamental importance for our body cells to function properly. Today, our diets have reversed this ratio to about 6 sodium to 1 potassium.

Owner's Manual: Avoid added salt in cooking, in processed foods, and at the table.

Healthy Fatty Acid Profile

All the evidence we have seen indicates that the human organism should be eating fat only moderately. A rough guideline suggests that maximum intake should not exceed 20 percent of calories from all sources. However, the fat that we do eat should be of specific kinds. In Chapter 3, we looked into the vital role that the various fatty acids play in manipulating our biochemistry. There are twenty-five different fatty acids and most play no significant part in human nutrition. However, a handful that should not be there create havoc with the body's workings, and some that we desperately need are absent. The only fatty acids that we need to be consuming are omega-3 oils and omega-6 oils. Furthermore, they should be in the ideal ratio of 1 to 1—the closer you can get to this ratio, the better.

Depending on what creature or plant they come from, some particular fatty acids are readily absorbed by the body, and these are said to be "bioavailable." There are other foods that contain unsafe fatty acids, but these are not bioavailable and thus are less likely to be absorbed by the body. We will make use of this knowledge when deciding what foods are safe and which are harmful. This can produce surprising results that are sometimes contrary to what a simplistic analysis of their fatty acid composition might indicate.

Owner's Manual: Eat no more than 20 percent of calories as fat/oil. Focus on consumption of bioavailable omega-3 fatty acids, reduce consumption of bioavailable omega-6 fatty acids, and avoid foods with bioavailable "bad" fatty acids.

High Micronutrient Content

When we talk about micronutrients, we include not only all the familiar vitamins and minerals, but also the thousands of "background" micronutrients. These are found predominantly in non-starchy plant food. We realize that many diseases, vague ills, and premature aging are symptoms of micronutrient deficiency. Today, micronutrient-poor starchy plant foods such as grains, rice, and potatoes have crowded out micronutrient-rich non-starchy plant foods. We saw how, in the Savanna Model, our ancient food supply contained both high concentrations and high volumes of micronutrients. This is the situation we need to return to today.

Owner's Manual: Consume only non-starchy plant food and conforming fruits and vegetables.

Low Plant Poison (Anti-nutrient) Levels

Earlier, we revealed that many of our commonly consumed foods contain background levels of plant poisons, or "anti-nutrients." Our ancestral diet did not contain such foods and our bodies do not know how to deal with them. We will all find better vitality and health when we eliminate such foods from our diets.

Owner's Manual: Avoid grains, legumes, and potatoes, which contain anti-nutrients.

Low Antigen Content

Many of our commonly consumed foods contain harmful doses of immune system saboteurs, or "antigens." Our ancestral diet did not contain such foods—and our bodies do not know how to deal with them. We need to eliminate these foods from our diet.

Owner's Manual: Avoid dairy and grains, which contain antigens.

Feel Hungry Regularly

On the condition that they are all still living and eating in their traditional states, the San, Japanese, Okinawans, and Cretans are slim people (see Appendix A on page 162). They eat sparingly and they often feel hungry, yet these peoples are all remarkable for their good health and longevity. The slimmer you are (without being emaciated), the longer you are likely to live and the less disease you will suffer. All the evidence points to this factor as being an essential characteristic of a healthy, naturally adapted lifestyle.

However, even if we cannot be skinny, there is a halfway house we should try to reach to make sure that the blood sugar control machinery functions smoothly. Insulin is the sugar "locking-up" hormone and its counterpart, glucagon, is the sugar "unlocking" hormone. Glucagon instructs fat cells to convert fat into sugar and release it into the bloodstream. Lack of use often atrophies this vital function of our biochemistry. Blood sugar levels have to be low and maintained low for the glucagon mechanism to swing into action. That means feeling hungry for about thirty minutes on a regular basis. Older people will remember that this happened several times a day before a main meal. Today, we do not allow ourselves the chance to be hungry; if people feel even slightly hungry, there is always a sugar-boosting snack within easy reach.

Owner's Manual: Feel hungry for thirty minutes two or three times a day.

Overview of Implementation

When we put together these criteria with what we know about certain groups of foods, these are the broad outlines for implementation of the Savanna Model.

- Consume a weight of conforming colored plant food that is about three times the weight of conforming protein-rich food. This means consuming an abundance of non-starchy, colored plant foods and low-glycemic fruits, while consuming protein-rich foods modestly.

- Eliminate salt added at the table and in processing or cooking.

- Consume fats and oils sparingly. In addition, eliminate saturated fats in non-conforming foods, drastically curtail omega-6 oils, and boost consumption of omega-3 oils.

- Eliminate grains in all their forms.

- Eliminate potato in all its forms.

- Eliminate dairy products in all their forms.

- Eliminate processed foods.

- Feel hungry for at least thirty minutes two or three times a day.

The 80-15-5 Rule

All this might seem daunting, but you don't have to be perfect; the healthy body is quite resilient and it can cope with some disharmony. So we often talk of the 80-15-5 rule: If 80 percent of your diet and lifestyle choices are spot-on, then 15 percent can be a little off, and the remaining 5 percent is reserved for the real lapses and special occasions, such as when it is Thanksgiving, a wedding anniversary, and so forth. Of course, if you are fighting a life-threatening disease, then you have to decide who wins—you or the disease.

Next, we will discover which are the "conforming" plant foods and "conforming" protein-rich foods that are readily available to us today. We will answer the challenge of how to adapt the Savanna Model to the food supply in the modern world. The choices are not always as obvious as we might think.

THE SAVANNA MODEL TODAY

For this information to be useful, we need to relate it to our everyday lives. Our Pleistocene ancestors had incredible jungle survival skills, and we have to develop the same level of skill for survival in the supermarket jungle. There is not a single food that we eat today that our forager forebears would have recognized in the African savanna. So, for example, even when we talk in broad terms about eating fruits, our ancestors' fruits were different species—with somewhat different nutrient profiles—from our apples, oranges, and pears today. That is why we have to be well-informed about everything we eat and why we go into some detail to explain how to make wise food choices.

We will categorize foods according to how closely they conform to the Savanna Model. The classification is based on a traffic light system: Green means "Go," Amber (yellow) means "Caution," and Red means "Stop." We introduce finer gradations, such as "Green-Amber," which means "Go, but proceed with caution." Green-Green means "Go-Go!"—these are superfoods which are particularly healthful. The classification system breaks down as follows:

- **Green-Green:** *Perfect*—in perfect conformity with the Savanna Model.

- **Green:** *Conforming*—in close conformity with the Savanna Model.

- **Green-Amber:** *Comfort Zone*—within the margin of tolerance for everyday consumption by a healthy person.

- **Amber:** *Slight Lapse*—acceptable for a healthy person to consume on a regular basis, provided the rest of the diet is conforming.

- **Amber-Red:** *Modest Lapse*—acceptable for a healthy person to consume on an occasional basis, provided the rest of the eating pattern is conforming.

- **Red:** *Bad Lapse*—not acceptable; avoid.

The following sections will break down the eating pattern into several food groups, and name those foods that are safe and tolerable for us to eat.

Food Group 1—Grains and Seeds

In this work, we use the common meanings for grains and seeds:

Seeds are the small, hard kernels of flowering plants that, when planted in the ground, will germinate and grow into a new plant. Examples are flaxseed, sesame seed, hemp seed, and rapeseed (canola).

Grains are just one kind of seed. They are seeds of grasses. Examples are wheat, barley, rice, and corn (maize). In this work, we use the word "seed" to cover everything *except* "grains."

This is the great shock to conventional nutritional ideas: Grains are not the best thing since sliced bread! Grains are not a natural human food and they do nasty things to our bodies. They cause the human organism a number of problems, from unhealthy blood-sugar spikes to the contribution of plant toxins (anti-nutrients) and immune system depressors (antigens). They are poor in nutrients and crowd out more nutritious foods.

Grains include wheat, rice, rye, barley, and oats, as well as the "pseudo" grains such as amaranth and quinoa, and "heirloom" or "heritage" grains such as einkorn and emmer wheat. We also include the products made from grains: Bread, spaghetti, pizza, croissants, cookies, and so on.

In making this blanket condemnation, we hear protests in the background. What about whole grains? What about oats, which the manufacturers sell as "lowering cholesterol"? The reality is that marketing forces have distorted the true perspective. Whole grains may contain useful nutrients, such as wheat germ, but they are just as glycemic, and the bran contains even more anti-nutrients and antigens.

Oats, of all the grains, contain rather more soluble fiber than average, a quality that manufacturers promote as cholesterol-reducing and therefore heart-healthy. This, nevertheless, is not a valid argument: They are still glycemic, contain anti-nutrients and antigens, and are deficient in micronutrients. Oats are no alternative to proper plant food, like lettuce and avocado.

The human diet is far better off without any cereals and their products. However, not all grains have all the same drawbacks and the way they are prepared modifies, for better or for worse, these drawbacks. The criteria used to categorize the foods in the Grains Group are: Their effect on blood sugar surges, their anti-nutrient content, their gluten content, and their allergen content. They are all classified as "Red" in some degree. The purist will not have them in the house.

FOOD GROUP 1   GRAINS & SEEDS

GREEN-GREEN

SEEDS & SEED PRODUCTS chia seed, butter, flour	flaxseed butter flaxseed flour	hempseed butter hempseed flour

AMBER

SEEDS & SEED PRODUCTS pumpkin seed	sesame seed tahini (sesame butter)	

AMBER-RED

GRAINS barley, pearl **GRAIN PRODUCTS** **Bakery** black bread porridge	pumpernickel vollkornbrot **Breakfast Cereals** all bran oatmeal	**Pasta** all, including: gnocchi, lasagna, linguine, macaroni, noodles, spaghetti

RED

GRAINS barley, cracked bulgur wheat corn (maize) corn on the cob oats and oat bran rice—all types rye sweet corn (mature) wheat **GRAIN PRODUCTS** **Bakery** all, including: bagel, baguette, rye, white bread, wholewheat bread buns, generally	cakes cookies crackers, water croissant Danish pastry gateaux muffin pastry, generally pizza, all kinds pretzels tarts **Breakfast Cereals** bran cereals Cheerios corn flakes hominy	muesli Rice Krispies Shredded Wheat Weetabix **Sundry** corn starch couscous pancakes pie crust popcorn rice cakes rice pudding semolina waffles

Food Group 2—Starchy Vegetables

Starchy plant foods are high-glycemic (they cause unhealthy blood sugar surges), and for this reason alone, you should avoid them. In addition, the most prominent of these foods in the Western diet, potatoes, are exceptionally bad for you: They are not only highly glycemic, they are highly insulinemic and also contain "background" poisons. Other starchy plants are parsnip and rutabaga, and it is best to go easy on them, too.

There are some vegetables that are sugary, notably carrots and beets (beetroot). For this reason, they are included with the starchy vegetables. The glycemic index of carrots can vary considerably, but if they are raw and mature, they have only a modest impact on blood sugar levels. This is where we deploy the concept of glycemic load. Carrots have a low calorie density, so you have to eat quite a lot before triggering a glycemic reaction. Depending on age and a variety of factors, including those to do with the vagaries of climate and soil, they can be more or less glycemic. Therefore, because we want to take in their good micronutrients and fibers, we allow the carrot a small place in our diet. Be wary, though, of carrot juice: It is more glycemic than the raw, unprocessed vegetable. Beets also are quite glycemic, but since they are rich in certain antioxidants, they just creep into the "Amber" category.

FOOD GROUP 2	VEGETABLES, STARCHY	
GREEN-AMBER		
Vegetables beets, raw	carrot, raw, mature	
AMBER		
Vegetables beets, red (beetroot)	carrot, baby carrot, cooked	pumpkin yam (Dioscorea)
AMBER-RED		
Vegetables parsnip	rutabaga (swede) sweet potato	tapioca
RED		
Potatoes French fries	potato, baked potato, boiled	potato, chips potato, mashed

Food Group 3—Non-starchy Vegetables

With this group, we finally come in contact with foods that are in full conformity with the Savanna Model. Ideally, we would eat these raw. However, if you choose to cook, always employ the gentlest cooking methods.

Since we are recommending that you consume an abundance of conforming non-starchy, colored plant foods, what plant foods are "conforming"? They are foods that are low-glycemic, rich in micronutrients and fiber, and harmless with regard to anti-nutrients and antigens. Broadly, they include most salad foods, such as lettuce, onions, cucumber, radish, and mushrooms, and they also include colored vegetables, such as broccoli, green beans, bell peppers (sweet peppers), and Brussels sprouts. These are considered "Green-Green," "Green," and "Green-Amber." Under "Green-Green," we have separated out the vegetables that have the high concentrations of background micronutrients that our ancient ancestors delighted in. You can have unlimited consumption of these foods, and the ideal is up to two pounds (900 g) per day.

Note that we include "baby" sweet corn as a good salad vegetable. Unlike its mature form, the grains in baby corn have not yet formed and it is neither starchy nor glycemic. Tomatoes, because of their mild background anti-nutrients, only receive qualified approval in the "Green-Amber" category. Chili pepper and curry powder (particularly the "hot" variety) are to be used sparingly, if ever at all; they damage the colon and make it leaky. Sauerkraut and other pickles receive a poor rating because of their high salt content. Ketchup has several possible ratings. The best is our own Savanna Model recipe (see our companion cookbook *Paleo Harvest*). If not, speciality ketchups are commercially available, which use "safer" ingredients: Tomatoes, canola oil, and fructose.

We also include a meat substitute made from fungus known as "mycoprotein." The manufacturer, Quorn, makes it available either in its raw state as a kind of ground meat look-alike or made up into veggie burgers, frankfurters, and so on. Mycoprotein is by far the best meat substitute when compared to soy protein or wheat gluten protein (seitan). Mycoprotein has a medium protein content, on a par with eggs (about 12 g protein per 100 g).

FOOD GROUP 3 VEGETABLES, NON-STARCHY		
GREEN-GREEN		
Vegetables	cabbage, white	**Herbs**
beet greens	cauliflower	garlic
broccoli	kale	ginger
Brussels sprouts	Swiss chard	parsley
cabbage, red	turnip greens	

FOOD GROUP 3 VEGETABLES, NON-STARCHY *continued*

GREEN

Condiments
all other herbs
lemon juice
vinegar, all kinds

Meat Substitute
mycoprotein (Quorn)

Sauces and Dips
guacamole

Vegetables
alfalfa sprouts
artichoke
asparagus
avocado
bean sprouts

bell pepper
bok choy
celeriac
celery
chicory
coleslaw
cress
cucumber
egg plant
endive
fennel
garlic
green beans
Jerusalem artichoke
kohl rabi

leeks
lettuce
mushroom
okra
onion
palm heart
radish
spinach
sugar snap peas
summer squash (marrow)
sweet corn, baby
turnip
water chestnut
watercress
zucchini (courgette)

GREEN-AMBER

Condiments
mustard

Pickles
onions, pickled

Sauces
ketchup, reduced sugar,
reduced salt

Vegetables
tomatoes

AMBER

Condiments
curry, mild

Pickles
gherkins, low-salt
olives, rinsed

Sauces
salsa, mild
ketchup, regular

AMBER-RED

Condiments
curry, medium

Pickles
gherkins, salty
olives, salty

sauerkraut

Sauces
salsa, hot

RED

Condiments
chili pepper

curry, hot

Sauces
Tabasco

Food Group 4—Fruits

Fruits today have quite different nutritional characteristics to those of our ancestors of the African Pleistocene era. The most troubling difference lies in the sugar content: It is often high and it is often glycemic. Even if they are not glycemic, the fructose content can be at worrisome levels. Some sugars, like fructose, do not raise blood sugar levels, but in large quantities upset other aspects of our biochemistry (see "Fructose" section below). In other respects, fruits are generally a rich source of valuable micronutrients, so we need to prioritize which fruits to focus on.

Fructose

We have come a long way since the 1990s when dietitians thought that fructose, being kind to blood sugar levels, was the perfect answer to the mischief of table sugar. We now know that fructose has a dark side that is just as bad as table sugar.

Professor George Bray estimates that as long ago as 1997, the average American was consuming 60 g of fructose per day and rising. Researchers find that a diet high in fructose has drawbacks. By "high in fructose," they mean an intake of 100 g (20 teaspoons) per day. By today's standards, this is not so much. Many people can get to this level by drinking just four 12-ounce cans of cola. At this level of consumption, fructose undermines blood sugar control, provokes diarrhea and bloating, and drives up glucose intolerance, blood pressure, cholesterol, triglycerides, and insulin resistance. Much of these effects are caused by the way fructose interacts with an enzyme in the cells called ATP. (See inset "Fructose's ATP Effect" below.)

Recent studies[1] find that even moderate consumption of fructose by adolescents increases blood pressure, fasting glucose, insulin resistance, and inflam-

Fructose's ATP Effect

Why does fructose create such harm? One reason is the way the body processes it. The power plant in every cell relies on an enzyme called ATP. However, the conversion of fructose in the liver also requires ATP. Here lies the danger. If too much fructose is consumed, the excess fructose, by competing for ATP, drains it from its primary duty—of powering the cell.[2] One result of ATP depletion is increased inflammation and scarring in the liver. Another is boosted creation of fats, leading to fatty liver and increased production of uric acid. Too much uric acid is a factor in gout, high blood pressure, cardiovascular disease, type 2 diabetes, metabolic syndrome, and a form of kidney stones. Much mischief, therefore, comes just from this aspect of overdosing on fructose.

matory cytokines; they have lower HDL ("good") cholesterol and adiponectin, a hormone which regulates (amongst many things) glucose and fatty acid oxygenation; they also are more likely to have internal belly fat, a risk factor for cardiovascular disease and diabetes.

A fructose-rich diet has many harmful consequences:

- In pregnant women, fructose programs the fetus for hypertension, insulin resistance, and obesity as an adult.[3] Moreover, this effect is transmitted down the generations.

- It predisposes male offspring to autism.[4]

- In a study on rats, fructose was found to sabotage learning and memory.[5]

- In monkeys, fructose consumption caused liver damage that was more than doubled over six weeks.[6]

- It is a principal driver of type 2 diabetes in people.[7]

- In mice, fructose is more toxic than table sugar. It reduces fitness and survival.[8]

- It contributes to weight gain, slows physical activity, and increases body fat.[9]

- It leads to uncontrolled growth of cardiomyocytes (heart cells), a factor in heart disease.[10]

- It undermines the brain's ability to heal after injury—at least in rats.[11]

Finally, after this litany of harms, let us not forget that fructose is empty calories—the more you consume, the more likely you are to get fat.

Fructose was always scarce in our ancestral diet, so the body's only reflex is to keep eating it for as long as supplies are available. So, just as with fat and salt, the body has never had to develop a reflex which says: "Enough!". Now, in the modern world of fructose abundance, that is why we have to take control of fructose intake for ourselves.

What does this mean? Professor Robert Lustig of University of California, San Francisco, says we can make an exception for fruits. However, I believe we need to be cautious and try to work with low-fructose (and low-glycemic) varieties. See the table "Food Group 4—Fruits" on page 66.

Other forms of added fructose need to be stripped out of the diet with just the same zeal as for table sugar itself. Perhaps the worst culprits are carbonated beverages, but they are closely followed by table sugar, high-glucose syrup, and high fructose corn syrup (HCFS) in a huge variety of processed foods. Be alert— we shouldn't be eating them anyway! In the words of Professor Bray, "Fructose, by any other name, is a health hazard."[12]

Low-Glycemic Fruits

Fruits that are both low-glycemic and low-sugar are "good" to eat without restriction, and so have been placed in the "Green" category in the table below. Fruits in this category include gooseberry and raspberry. There are other low-glycemic fruits, such as cherries, which nevertheless have a significant content of various sugars. There is not a direct correlation between sugar content and glycemic index (this was the great insight of David Jenkins; see page 21). You should go easy on these fruits if your doctor is asking you to restrict your intake of fructose or glucose.

Borderline-Glycemic Fruits

These fruits tend not only to be relatively glycemic, but they also often have a correspondingly high sugar content. It is good to incorporate them into the daily diet because of their nutrient content, but keep their consumption modest. Examples are apple, pear, orange, and strawberry.

High-Glycemic Fruits

Many fruits, often of tropical origin, are high-glycemic. They are not pariahs, but we should not go out of our way to obtain them. If you find a morsel or two in your fruit salad, swallow it down; it won't poison you. But do not consume these regularly or copiously. Examples are watermelon, pineapple, and ripe banana.

The fruits classified as "Green" are mostly low-sugar berries; they are often exceptionally good sources of antioxidants, too. Cranberries, in the raw state, are extremely nutritious and low in sugar. Unfortunately, they are so astringent that they can make the lips pucker up. For this reason, cranberries are often heavily dosed with sugar, either as a jelly or stewed in sugar. This process converts a great fruit into a bad one. Bananas become more sugary as they ripen; the greener you can stand them, the better.

You should treat dried fruit (raisins, currants, dates, figs, apricots, peaches, etc.) as sugars. The drying process destroys some of the micronutrients, so in no way can dried fruit be a substitute for the fresh variety. In addition, we do not recommend that you liquidize fruits. Juicing, pasteurizing, concentrating, and reconstituting are processes that destroy the nature and utility of the natural fibers, strip out the nutrients, and increase the glycemic index.

FOOD GROUP 4 FRUITS		
GREEN LOW-FRUCTOSE, LOW GLYCEMIC INDEX		
bilberry	cranberry, fresh,	elderberry
blackberry	unsweetened	gooseberry

FOOD GROUP 4 FRUITS *continued*

GREEN LOW-FRUCTOSE, LOW GLYCEMIC INDEX *continued*

grapefruit	raspberry	**Vegetable-fruits**
lemon	redcurrants	avocado
nectarine	strawberry, wild	
pomelo	whitecurrant	

GREEN-AMBER LOW-FRUCTOSE, BORDERLINE GLYCEMIC INDEX

banana, unripe (green)	peach	**Vegetable-fruits**
blueberry	plum	tomato
guava	strawberry, cultivated	
orange	tangerine	

AMBER LOW-FRUCTOSE, HIGH GLYCEMIC INDEX

apricot, fresh	melon, cantaloupe	pineapple
kiwi	melon, horned	watermelon

AMBER MEDIUM-FRUCTOSE, LOW GLYCEMIC INDEX

blackcurrants	cherries	papaya

AMBER-RED HIGH-FRUCTOSE, BORDERLINE GLYCEMIC INDEX

apples	dates, raw	pears
cranberries, sweetened	lychees	pomegranate

RED-AMBER HIGH-FRUCTOSE, HIGH GLYCEMIC INDEX

banana (ripe)	apricots, dried	prickly pear
custard apple	grapes	prunes
dates, dried	mango	raisins
figs, dried	persimmon (kaki, sharon)	sultanas

Food Group 5—Dairy Products

Dairy products are a biochemical disaster for the human organism—we do not have the digestive enzymes to assimilate them properly and they contain a range of compounds that bring bad health. Chief among them is lactose (which is highly allergenic), but we can also cite dairy fats (saturated and artery-clogging) and dairy proteins (allergenic and cholesterol-disrupting). Refer back to

Chapter 3 for more information on these allergens. Whether "raw" or processed, from cows or goats, whether turned into yogurt or cheese, dairy products are all classified in various degrees of "Red."

Cheese lovers have a slight consolation, as cheese is the least harmful of dairy products: Cheeses have less lactose and, seemingly, their bad fats are not readily absorbed by the body. Cheese can be consumed modestly on the rare occasion. When you commit this offense against the Savanna Model, make sure that it is worth it—that the cheese is a really good one—and savor every nibble slowly, spreading it carefully around the palate. However, do not use a platform of bread or cracker, unless it is made from a Paleo-conforming recipe. (See *Paleo Harvest* cookbook in the Resources, and sample recipes in Appendix B.)

FOOD GROUP 5 DAIRY		
AMBER-RED		
Milk Products cheeses, all kinds		
RED		
Milk Products buttermilk ice cream ice cream, low-fat milk, buffalo	milk, cow's, condensed milk, cow's, evaporated milk, cow's, full fat milk, cow's, skimmed milk, goat's	milk, sheep's whey yogurt, full fat yogurt, reduced fat yogurt, all varieties

Food Group 6—Meat, Poultry, Eggs, and Fish

Animal matter has formed a moderate part of the human diet for an evolutionarily significant part of human history. As we have seen, the type of animal matter was rather different. In the sections below, we make judgments about the animal matter available to us today. The chief criterion is the fatty acid profile—the quantity of fat and the types of fatty acids. In addition, some variety meats (such as offal, the organ meats) can contain unhealthy amounts of some substances (e.g., iron and vitamin A, which can build up excessively in the liver).

Farm Meat

Common farm meats, such as beef, pork, and lamb, have become problem foods. The difficulty is their high fat content and the harmful nature of the fat. Stockbreeders are beginning to work on improving the nutritional nature of their herds, but for now, we are better off avoiding these meats and everything that is made from them. An occasional exception can be made for beef: Its saturated fat is a) partly stearic acid, which the body readily converts into safe oleic acid (olive oil) and, b) less bioavailable (i.e., less readily absorbed by the body) because of where it is positioned on the triglyceride molecule. Likewise, the goat is naturally very low in fat and is, indeed, fully Savanna Model conforming.

Wild Game

In most instances, meat from various wild creatures has a conforming fatty acid profile. Truly wild game that feeds off what it finds in its natural habitat is an approved animal matter and is fine to consume in moderation. It will be low-fat and should have a good fatty acid profile. This includes wild boar, moose, caribou, and bison.

Variety Meats (Offal)

Our Pleistocene ancestors ate all parts of a slain animal, but this did not happen all that often. Many of the internal organs have wildly varying nutrient composition, depending on a number of factors: What the animal ate recently, how it was raised, and even its state of health. It is difficult, therefore, to generalize about variety meats. They are usually rich in micronutrients not found in such high concentrations in other sources. Variety meats are normally all right to consume in moderate quantities on an occasional basis.

Kidney, tripe, and liver are low-fat meats, but liver in particular is heavily loaded with vitamin A and arachidonic acid (an omega-6 fatty acid that can cause inflammation), both of which are harmful in high doses; you should consume it with caution. Tongue, heart, and brains are high-fat meats, with much of the fat saturated, and brains are particularly rich in cholesterol; eat these only occasionally.

Not many Americans eat variety meats as it is, but they are still consuming them without even realizing it. That is because meatpackers disguise them as salami, hot dogs, luncheon meats, and sausage. These products should definitely be avoided because they are high-fat (most of it unhealthy), salty, and often doctored with sulfur compounds to preserve them.

Exotic Animal Matter

This category includes such creatures as alligator, ostrich, emu, kangaroo, frogs' legs, and escargots (snails). All correspond very well to the kind of animal matter that our Pleistocene ancestors ate all the time. Other exotic foods are making their appearance, particularly bush tucker from Australia, which corresponds to the food traditionally eaten by the Australian Aboriginal. My wife and I have sat down with Aborigines in Central Australia to eat one of their delicacies, the witchety grub. Lightly roasted in the embers of a fire, this three-inch-long caterpillar tastes rather like sweet corn.

Poultry (Farm and Wild)

The low-fat parts of farm fowl, such as skinless chicken and turkey breast, are good in modest quantities. You should reduce consumption of other parts as much as possible. All parts of duck and goose are fine. Wild birds such as pheasant, grouse, and pigeon are fully conforming.

Eggs

Our Pleistocene forebears consumed all kinds of eggs: Ostrich, bustard, duck, and anything else they could find. Hen's eggs come close, with a proviso—seek out eggs that are rich in omega-3 oils, and it is preferable if they are also free-range and organic. Duck, turkey, quail, and goose eggs are good, too. Industrially produced eggs are a poor substitute and should not be consumed on a regular basis.

Seafood

All seafood is an acceptable component of the Savanna Model feeding pattern. The "oily fish," rich in omega-3 oils, are best, such as wild salmon, sardines, herring, and mackerel. Other fish and shellfish have an excellent essential fatty acid profile and are also good.

FOOD GROUP 6 MEAT, POULTRY, EGGS, AND FISH		
GREEN-GREEN		
Eggs	mackerel	**Fish, shellfish**
eggs, omega-3	salmon	clam
Fish, finfish	sardine	oysters
herring	trout	shrimp
	tuna	squid
GREEN		
Eggs	caviar	sea bass
all other eggs, including:	cod	sea bream
eggs, chicken	eel	shark
eggs, duck	haddock	skate
eggs, goose	halibut	swordfish
eggs, quail	monkfish	turbot
eggs, turkey	pike	**Fish, shellfish**
Fish, finfish	pollock	all shellfish, including:
all other fish, including:	roe	calamari
carp	roughy, orange	crab

FOOD GROUP 6   MEAT, POULTRY, EGGS, AND FISH *continued*

GREEN *continued*

crayfish

cuttlefish

lobster

mussels

octopus

prawns

scallop

whelks

Meat, exotic

crocodile

escargots (snails)

frogs' legs

turtle

Meat, farmed

goat

rabbit

Meat, game

bison

boar, wild

buffalo

caribou

deer (venison)

elk

horse

moose

Meat, offal

kidney

tripe

Poultry, farmed

chicken, breast, skinless

duck

emu

goose

ostrich

turkey, breast, skinless

Poultry, wild

duck, wild

goose, wild

partridge

pheasant

pigeon

quail

AMBER

Meat, farmed

beef, all kinds

beef, spare ribs

beef, steaks

Meat, offal

brains

heart

liver

thymus

tongue

AMBER-RED

Meat, farmed

veal

Poultry, farmed

chicken, buffalo wings

chicken, drumstick

chicken, wings

turkey, drumstick

turkey, wings

RED

Meat, farmed

lamb, all kinds

lamb, chops

lamb, leg

pork, all kinds

pork, bacon

pork, chops

pork, ham

pork, leg

Meat, processed

beef burger

bologna

bratwurst

cold meats

frankfurter

hamburger

lunch meat

meat paste

pate de foie gras

salami

sausage

Spam

Food Group 7—Legumes

Legumes are newcomers to the human diet and there are major drawbacks to consuming them: The body is not equipped to handle their plant poisons (anti-nutrients) and antigens. Only from time to time may you include a moderate portion of legumes in your diet; the purist will avoid them altogether. Examples of legumes are lentils, beans, and peanuts. Peas are legumes but are a slightly different case: They contain fewer anti-nutrients, but on the other hand, they are starchy and glycemic. In addition, we single out the soybean for special mention because of its false reputation as a miracle food—avoid soy and all its products (tofu, soy protein burgers, tofu-substitute yogurts, and so on).

FOOD GROUP 7 LEGUMES		
AMBER-RED		
Legume Products	hummus (chickpea dip)	peas
beans, baked, low-sugar and low-salt	noodles, Chinese bean	
RED		
Beans, all, including:	beans, pinto	**Soy, all, including:**
beans, adzuki	beans, refried	soy, bean
beans, baked, canned	beans, white	soy, cheese substitute
beans, broad	chickpeas (garbanzo)	soy, meat substitute
beans, fava	lentils, green	soy, milk substitute
beans, garbanzo	lentils, red	soy, protein
beans, haricot	peanut butter	soy, tofu
beans, kidney	peanuts	soy, yogurt substitute
beans, mung	peas, mushy	vetch
beans, navy	pease pudding	

Food Group 8—Nuts

Nuts are a natural food for humans to be consuming. All tree nuts are generally fine. Examples are walnuts, almonds, Brazil nuts, and filberts. However, chestnuts, coconut, and peanuts do not fit into this tree nut category. Chestnuts are mainly starch and so are included in the starchy vegetable group; coconuts are mainly oil and are included in the fats and oils group. Peanuts are *not* nuts; they are a legume and are included in the previous legume group.

Nuts should be raw and fresh. Regrettably, food manufacturers usually roast and salt nuts to improve shelf life and taste. However, this destroys useful nutrients and the salt is an unwelcome burden to the diet. Around half the weight of a nut is oil, much of it omega-6 fatty acids. Nuts are therefore calorie-dense and tend to upset the omega-3 to omega-6 balance. For these reasons, nuts should be consumed in moderation. Those classified "Green-Green" have a high omega-3 content. We make special mention of walnuts, which have the exceptional property of being rich in omega-3 oil. However, it is essential that the walnuts be fresh, because their omega-3 oil turns rancid very easily and becomes an oxidized fat particularly harmful to cardiovascular health.

FOOD GROUP 8 NUTS		
GREEN-GREEN		
Tree Nuts		
walnut		
GREEN		
Tree Nuts	filbert (hazelnut, cobnut)	pistachio
almond	macadamia	**Note:** All nuts must be
brazil	pecan	fresh, raw, and unsalted.
cashew	pine	

Food Group 9—Fats and Oils

In nature, fats and oils do not occur on their own: They are always part of something else. The Bushman could not eat the mongongo oil without eating the nut; he could not eat the animal fat without eating the animal. Fats and oils in their separated state are in a very concentrated form and therefore more potent. That is why they should always be treated with caution.

As a rule of thumb, oils that are solid at room temperature are suspect, as they are almost certainly unhealthy saturated fats. Examples are butter, lard (including bacon fat), and tallow (beef and sheep fat). Artificial saturated fats are equally unhealthy, such as trans fats and hydrogenated fats. They are present in many processed foods and in margarines and spreads. In other words, all fats should be avoided.

The general injunction is to consume oils sparingly. We should focus on omega-3 oils. A prime example is canola (rapeseed) oil, which is readily available in supermarkets. However, we recommend going for cold-pressed, organic canola oil, if possible. Flaxseed oil has the highest concentrations of omega-3s and is preferred if you can afford it. The oil is fragile and needs to be kept in the refrigerator and consumed within a few weeks. Other options are hempseed oil and walnut oil (make sure it is not made from roasted walnuts).

All these omega-3 oils should only be used cold—in a salad dressing, for example. Omega-3 oils do not resist heat very well and the oil oxidizes and becomes toxic. If you need to heat the oil for cooking, then a monounsaturated (and thus inert) oil is best. Canola oil can fit the bill since its omega-3 content will withstand modest temperatures up to 340°F. We advise that cooking should never exceed this temperature anyway, but if it does, then olive oil is safest to use.

The human organism also needs a second class of oil, the omega-6s, in a balanced ratio with the omega-3s. The trouble in the modern diet is that omega-6 vegetable oils are in everything and thus overwhelm our omega-3 consumption. We must therefore avoid any unnecessary intake. For this reason, you should strictly avoid knowingly consuming omega-6 oils, such as sunflower oil, safflower oil, peanut oil, and corn oil.

The criteria we have used in our classification are: Omega-3 content; omega-6 to omega-3 ratio; and presence of harmful fatty acids, such as palmitic acid and myristic acid. In addition, we have taken into account the bioavailability of the "good" fatty acids and the "bad" fatty acids. That is to say, the position of these fatty acids on the glycerol molecule is an important factor. In this way, for example, cocoa butter and coconut oil and butter have a more favorable category than a simple examination of their saturated fat content would have predicted. In all cases, fats and oils should be consumed with restraint. We have included mayonnaise and spreads, but it makes a big difference which oils they are made from. Check the labels and reject products that are "Amber-Red" or "Red." Watch out for hydrogenated fats in spreads and all kinds of processed foods.

FOOD GROUP 9   FATS AND OILS

GREEN-GREEN

Fish Oils	sardine oil	**Plant Oils**
all fish oil, including:	**Marine oils**	canola (rapeseed) oil
cod liver oil	all marine oils, including:	flaxseed oil
herring oil	seal oil	hemp oil
menhaden oil	whale oil	
salmon oil		

GREEN

Plant Oils	mayonnaise, olive oil	spread, olive oil (check the ingredients)
almond cream	olive oil	walnut oil
mayonnaise, canola	spread, canola (check the ingredients)	

FOOD GROUP 9 FATS AND OILS *continued*		
GREEN-AMBER		
Animal Fats	**Plant Oils**	coconut oil
duck fat	cocoa butter	sesame oil
goose fat	coconut butter	soybean oil
	coconut cream	
AMBER-RED		
Animal Fats	**Plant Oils**	peanut oil
tallow (beef fat)	corn oil	safflower oil
	mayonnaise, lite	spread, not "Green"
	mayonnaise, not "Green"	sunflower oil
RED		
Animal Fats	lard (pork fat)	margarine
butter	shortening	palm oil
cream	**Plant Oils**	trans fats, all
drippings	hydrogenated oil, all	

Food Group 10—Sugars and Sweeteners

Sweet-tasting foods were a rarity in our ancestral diet. Consumption of any of these items should be restrained. The various sweetnesses available to us today fall into three main categories: High-glycemic sugars, low-glycemic sugars, and intense (artificial) sweeteners.

High-glycemic Sugars

We have seen how most sugars—e.g., the high-glycemic ones such as table sugar—and most confectionary are harmful for us. They must be ruthlessly removed from the diet. More surprising for many of you is that the "natural" sugars, honey and maple syrup, are to be treated with caution. Some dried fruits have high sugar content and are highly glycemic; for example, dried figs, dried dates, sultanas, and dried apricots. They should be avoided.

Low-glycemic Sugars

Low-glycemic sugars include polyols and fructose.

Polyols (sugar alcohols). These are sweet-tasting dietary fibers of vegetable origin. Examples are sorbitol, erythritol, and xylitol. They are white and crystalline, like table sugar; they have similar levels of sweetness. They are absorbed to a greater or lesser extent in the digestive tract, partly by digestion, partly by gut bacteria. Depending on the degree of absorption, they have a higher or lower caloric value. For example, xylitol yields about 10 calories per teaspoon, but erythritol has zero calories (it is not absorbed at all). This compares to table sugar, at 15 calories per teaspoon.

In as much as they are dietary fibers, polyols feed good gut bacteria and so improve colon health. Xylitol, in addition, has been found to improve oral health[13]—that is why it is a valuable component of sugar-free chewing gum.

Some of the polyols can create temporary flatulence, which passes off once the subject is habituated. In spite of this mild drawback, when it comes to finding a substitute for table sugar, the various polyols are our favored candidates.

Fructose. A second class of low-glycemic sugars is based on fructose, a naturally occurring, low-glycemic sugar. However, as explained earlier (page 64), fructose for other reasons has become a health menace. So, although fructose itself is available in many supermarkets and health food stores, we do not recommend it. Fructose is present to a greater or lesser degree in honey. That is why, depending on which flower the honey comes from, the honey changes class.

The sugar from the agave plant is almost entirely fructose. Although it has a very low glycemic index, it cannot be recommended because of its fructose content.

In contrast, "high fructose corn syrup" is a misnomer. It has a composition very similar to table sugar and is just as glycemic.

The take-home message on fructose and fructose-containing products is that their consumption should be eliminated. With regard to fruits, we recommend focusing on the low-fructose, low-glycemic varieties. They are categorized "Green" in the Fruit table (see page 66).

Intense Sweeteners

What about intense (artificial) sweeteners such as aspartame, saccharine, sucralose, and so forth? In the past, we took a fairly relaxed attitude toward them on the principle that, when compared to table sugar, they appeared to be the lesser of two evils. However, there are two major drawbacks that have emerged in recent years:

• *The "cephalic phase insulin response."* This is where the brain, stimulated by sweet taste, anticipates the arrival of a blood sugar surge and so secretes a pulse of insulin. But with intense sweeteners, there is no blood sugar increase, the insulin surge is in vain, and only serves to create mischief and sugar cravings.[14]

● *Major alterations for the worse in gut bacteria.* The consumption of sucralose (Splenda), aspartame (Equal, Canderel), and especially saccharin (Sweet'n Low), causes an overgrowth of a particular profile of "bad" bacteria in the gut.[15] This leads to a number of mischiefs—especially a state of "glucose intolerance." Another study showed that sucralose halves the amount of good bacteria in the gut, boosts weight gain, and interferes with medications.[16] Apart from reducing the amount of *good* bacteria in the intestines by 50 percent, sucralose increased the acidity of the colon, which encourages the overgrowth of *bad* bacteria. These effects remained even after sucralose consumption had been discontinued for twelve weeks.

As for the natural sweetener, stevia, we know little about its effects, either good or bad. Most studies focus on potential benefits, such as its anti-diabetic, anti-microbial, and antioxidant properties. However, one study finds that it is potentially an endocrine disruptor; that is, it messes with hormones. Most notably, it boosts progesterone production which, in turn, interferes with sperm cells.[17] With regard to stevia's effect on gut bacteria, as of writing, there are no studies and we simply don't know yet.

My view on intense, artificial sweeteners is that they should be strictly avoided. With regard to stevia, the jury is out, but it seems wise to go easy on it, too.

Confectionary

Almost all confectionary (candy) is high in sugar and you should avoid it. However, all is not lost: Cocoa powder is low-glycemic. Chocolate that is made with a high percentage of cocoa solids (and therefore little sugar) is low-glycemic. Generally, if "cocoa solids" comes before sugar on the ingredients list, it is probably acceptable to eat. In the raw, natural state, cocoa is rich in the micronutrients known as flavanols. These flavonols are much vaunted for benefits such as reducing Alzheimer's risk,[18] LDL oxidation,[19] and inflammation.[20,21]

However, in the vast majority of cocoa and chocolate products, the flavanols are destroyed during the roasting, fermenting, and processing of the cocoa beans.[22] So, unless the product carries a credible flavonol claim, just eat very dark chocolate for the pleasure, not in the mistaken belief it will do you good, too!

Most other confectionary items are high-glycemic and devoid of useful nutrients; they usually contain bad fats and dairy as well—these belong to the dreaded "Red" column. Watch out for manufactured foods that claim to have "no sugar added." Often you are being duped: They can be sweetened with apple or grape juice concentrate, which are just as bad. However, some enterprising makers of diabetic chocolate (sweetened with polyols) have rebranded their chocolate as a "low-carb" or "diet" chocolate; these are fine in moderation.

FOOD GROUP 10   SUGARS & SWEETENERS

GREEN

Confectionary	Sugar Replacements	maltitol
chocolate, 85 percent	**(polyols)**	mannitol
cocoa solids	erythritol	sorbitol
	isomalt	xylitol
	lactitol	

GREEN-AMBER

Confectionary	Sweeteners	
chocolate, 75 percent	honey, max 8 tsp/day	
cocoa solids		

RED

Artificial Sweeteners	Nutri-Grain bar	cane sugar
acesulfame K	sweets, boiled	date sugar
aspartame	toffee	fruit sugars
saccharin		golden syrup
sucralose	**Sugar Aliases & Variants**	grape juice concentrate
Confectionary	dextrose	high fructose corn syrup
candies	galactose	invert sugar
chocolate (all except "Green"	glucose	malt
and "Green-Amber")	lactose	maple syrup
energy bars	levulose	molasses
fudge	maltodextrin	raw sugar
granola bar	maltose	sugar, brown
jelly beans	saccharose	sugar, Demerara
Life Savers	sucrose	sugar, icing, frosting
M&Ms	**Sweeteners**	sugar, table
Mars bar	apple juice concentrate	sugar, white
muesli bars	barley malt	treacle
	blackstrap molasses	

Food Group 11—Salt and Sodium

Salt needs to be ruthlessly eliminated from the diet. By far the biggest source is in processed foods; seemingly innocent foods like corn flakes contain more salt than does seawater. The examples are legion in manufactured food, so the best rule of thumb, as ever, is to avoid them altogether.

Our preoccupation is with the salt-to-potassium ratio. As we have previously described, salt has moved from being absent in the human diet to massively contaminating all aspects of our food supply. We are therefore obliged to adopt a strategy of avoiding all salt, whether incorporated in processed foods or added at the table or in cooking. These measures, together with the high consumption of plant foods (which are rich in potassium), will ensure that an optimum sodium-to-potassium ratio is maintained.

Here, we focus on external sources of salt. Not everyone realizes that garlic salt is plain salt with garlic flavoring; regular stock cubes are over 50 percent salt; soy sauce is just liquid salt fermented with soybeans. The "Amber" column contains some low-salt seasonings and also salt substitute.

Salt substitutes are based on potassium chloride rather than sodium chloride, since it has long been assumed that the problem is the *sodium.* However, a test with potassium chloride on salt-sensitive rats found that the *chloride* is also a part of the problem.[23]

There are dangers in over-consuming potassium chloride too, so although there often is little or no sodium in salt substitutes (check the ingredients label), they should only be consumed sparingly.

FOOD GROUP 11 SALT & SODIUM		
AMBER		
Sodium Products	stock cubes, low salt	yeast extract, Vegemite
salt substitute	yeast extract, Marmite	
AMBER-RED		
Sodium Products	seasoning, Maggi	stock cubes, Knorr
celery salt	soy sauce	stock cubes, Maggi
garlic salt	stock cubes, classic	stock cubes, Oxo
RED		
Sodium Products	Himalayan salt	rock salt
bicarbonate of soda	MSG (monosodium	sea salt
coarse salt	glutamate)	table salt

Food Group 12—Beverages

In Chapter 3, we cast doubt on the current preoccupation with guzzling water at every opportunity. The slogan "drink eight glasses a day" is a highly misleading piece of marketing by the mineral and bottled water companies. Other water manufacturers jumped on the bandwagon with so-called special property waters—mineralized, ionized, magnetized, polarized—a whole range of sales gimmicks to gull the public. We now live, quite falsely, in terror of not drinking enough water. Just know that if you follow the Savanna Model to the full, you will be getting four pints (64 oz) of water just from what you eat. The bottom line is that we need only drink when thirsty. By all means, drink bottled water, but water out of the tap is probably just as good.

Do not forget that tea, herbal teas, and coffee are valid thirst quenchers.[24] Cocoa is fine too, but make it with 100 percent cocoa powder (not chocolate mix) combined with water or almond milk. If you like, use a "Green" sweetener or honey.

Caffeine in coffee and tea is sometimes demonized in health circles. Nevertheless, almost all vegetation contains some caffeine and the body is quite capable of processing it without distress. It is only in certain plants that the concentrations reach mind-altering proportions. In modest quantities, caffeine can give increased mental performance and improve mood. Increasing the dosage can cause some unpleasant symptoms, such as irritability, anxiety, jitteriness, headaches, and insomnia. In addition, at higher doses, caffeine drives up insulin levels, increases insulin resistance, and makes it harder to lose weight.[25] However, the harmful effects of caffeine are reduced when it is present in tea or coffee. Scientists speculate that the other beneficial nutrients in these beverages compensate. Researchers have also found that a high consumption of micronutrient-rich plant food mitigates the harmful effects of caffeine on its own.

So, how quickly do we reach this safe limit? The average cup of American coffee contains 100 mg caffeine, whereas coffeehouse strength can be 180 mg per cup. The caffeine content of tea varies, but it averages about 40–50 mg per cup. There are also about 40 mg of caffeine in a 12-ounce can of cola. In a cocoa drink (2 teaspoons of pure cocoa powder), there are only 10 mg caffeine. Our view is that caffeine in modest amounts is well within the normal range for human consumption. (See "What Is 'Modest' Caffeine Consumption?" below.) For a 165-pound adult, that works out to four cups of American coffee per day or eight cups of tea. Be sensible about it, watch how your caffeine intake affects your

What Is "Modest" Caffeine Consumption?

A modest consumption of caffeine means about 2.75 mg per pound of body weight per day for the average adult. This works out to 450 mg for a 165-pound person. Children should be restricted to 1 mg per pound per day and reproductive-age women to 2.1 mg per pound per day. At these dosages, the drawbacks to caffeine use are minimal.[26]

mood, and avoid overdosing. If you are diabetic, caffeine in the form of moderate tea or coffee drinking might even be helpful.[27]

The "Amber-Red" and "Red" beverages are dominated by high-glycemic drinks, such as beer and colas, and by milk in its various forms. Milk is simply not human food and is harmful to our biochemistry. The milk of almonds (and other nuts) is a great alternative to regular milk, particularly in cookery. However, soy milk must be avoided. Fruit juices, even when freshly made, are glycemic—for this reason, they get the "Amber" classification. It is much better to eat the fruit itself. Watch out for tomato juice: Choose brands that are made from pure tomatoes and have no salt. Sugar-sweetened carbonated drinks and colas are high-glycemic and disrupt bone building.

Some alcohol drinks can be tolerated, but do not go out of your way to start consuming them if they are not already part of your diet. Beer is highly glycemic and potentially allergenic. Dry wine is acceptable and red wine is mildly healthful when consumed in moderation. One might be surprised at the moderate classification of spirits like gin and whiskey. Most spirits are all right, especially if diluted in a suitable, low-sugar mixer (for example, whiskey and soda; gin and diet tonic). Bear in mind that alcohol is empty calories and it disrupts your body's ability to burn fat, so you will struggle to lose weight if you consume alcohol.

FOOD GROUP 12 BEVERAGES

GREEN

almond milk	tea, black	water, mineral
cashew milk	tea, green	water, potable
cocoa, unsweetened	tea, herbal	water, purified
coconut milk	water, distilled	wine, dry, red

GREEN-AMBER

coffee, Americano	water, mineral, high sodium	wine, dry, white
grapefruit juice	wine, dry, champagne	sherry, dry
tomato juice, unsalted		

AMBER

apple juice, fresh	fruit juices, generally	soy milk substitute
cider, dry	orange juice, fresh	spirits: gin, whiskey, etc
cocoa, "Green" sweetener	pineapple juice, fresh	tomato juice, salted
coffee, espresso	port	wine, dessert
coffee, strong	sherry, sweet	wine, sweet

FOOD GROUP 12 BEVERAGES *continued*

AMBER-RED

beer, ale	beer, stout	liqueurs
beer, lager	cider	perry
beer, lite	fruit drinks	rice milk
beer, porter		

RED

cappuccino	colas, diet	milk, skimmed
chocolate drinks	fruit juices, sweetened	sodas, classic
coffee, made with milk	milk shake	sodas, non-cola, diet
colas, classic	milk, full-fat	yogurt drink

THE GOLDEN RULES

In order to live in harmony with the way nature intended, our eating pattern is the most important to get right. In my view, poor dietary habits are responsible for some 60 percent to 70 percent of what is going wrong with our health today. Moreover, this is one factor over which we can have total control!

In the sections below, you will find twelve basic rules for following this eating pattern, and four rules for other lifestyle factors to replicate the foragers' lifestyle as closely as possible.

Eating Pattern

A simple rule of thumb is to choose foods from the "Green" classes: "Green-Green," "Green," and "Green-Amber." Of these, Food Group 3 (Vegetables, Non-starchy) has no restrictions. "Green" classes in the other food groups should be consumed in controlled amounts.

1. The food to which as a species we are primarily adapted is plant food. Think big when planning volumes of salads and vegetables. Eat a minimum of one large mixed salad per day. Consume up to twelve ounces (350 g) of salads and twelve ounces (350 g) of colored vegetables per day. Put vegetables at the center of the plate ("Green" classes, Food Group 3).

2. Prefer raw vegetables to cooked. When cooking, use steaming, blanching, or stir-fry (sautéing) methods.

3. Eat fruit every day. Consume at least eight ounces (225 g) of fruit per day, but spread it out over several eating sessions ("Green" classes, Food Group 4).

4. The food to which we are secondarily adapted is animal matter. Think modest when planning servings of meat, poultry, eggs, and fish (Food Group 6).

5. Avoid red or fatty meat and their products ("Red" classes, Food Group 6).

6. Try to find the right balance at each meal between protein-rich foods (25 percent by weight) and plant foods (75 percent by weight). Concentrate on sources of "good" proteins ("Green" classes, Food Groups 6 and 8).

7. Avoid dairy products (Food Group 5).

8. Be frugal with fats and oils, even the "Green" classes. Never cook at high temperatures. Only bake or sauté at low temperatures—less than 320°F (160°C), although this may be a little higher for baking. Only use olive oil or canola (rapeseed) oil. Hot or cold, replace "Red" classes of fats and oils with "Green" classes such as olive oil, canola (rapeseed, colza) oil, hempseed oil, and flax oils (Food Group 9).

9. Drive down your salt and sodium intake. Processed foods, take-out, and restaurant meals are the worst offenders. Avoid using salt in cooking and at the table (Food Group 11).

10. Avoid industrial (processed) food. Be wary of anything that comes in a packet, can, jar, bottle, or box. Be wary of anything that has an ingredient label—read the fine print on the label and act on it!

11. Latest research indicates that your appetite will tell you to keep eating until your protein intake is satisfied. Aim to consume about 2 g of protein-rich foods per pound (0.5 kg) of body weight.

12. Feel hungry for at least thirty minutes two or three times a day.

Other Lifestyle Factors

Getting our food intake right is vital to good health—but we need to get the other lifestyle factors right too! If not, that works against the good we have done with a Paleo-conforming eating régime. Here, we summarize the main insights highlighted in Chapter 2.

1. **Physical Activity**

• Walk as much as you can. Aim for 10,000 steps per day, but the more, the better.

• Avoid sitting for too long. Get up from your desk every thirty minutes, stretch and walk forty to fifty paces around the office. Install a reminder in your smartphone or computer.

- Carry loads at every opportunity. You will avoid back problems later in life, especially if you start young. If you already have back problems, work with your health professional to integrate appropriate load-carrying into your life.

- Physical activity doesn't have to be particularly intense—although for able-bodied men, it is good to incorporate some aerobic activity every day.

- Women can get away with rather less physical activity than men.

2. **Environment and Stress**

Foragers, for all the challenges of life, were and are mentally well-adjusted.

- Try to choose opportunities to live and work where you can be exposed to green spaces. Even keeping house plants is helpful.

- Crowds are stressful. It is normal to want to "get away from it all" from time to time, so indulge that feeling.

- Most workplaces are unnatural environments. The more control you can exert over your livelihood, the better.

- Humans have a need to release the mind's pressure valve. It is normal to want to "lose oneself" at regular intervals. It can be done in a variety of ways, including meditation, dancing, music festivals, yoga, and the like.

- Humans feel most comfortable when they are part of a self-help social group of around fifty members. In our ancient ancestors' times, this would be the forager band which, in today's world, corresponds to an extended family. This represents a wide degree of "social connectedness," where the relationships are of moderate intensity. The Western world's nuclear family, where husband, wife, and two children live in intense relationship with each other, is actually unnatural and a recipe for stress. It is normal to enjoy being a member of a social group. Social groups can be of all kinds; the important aspect is social conviviality and the feeling that you are all mutually supportive, like in an extended family.

- There are so many other aspects of our daily lives that are out of sync with our psyches. Think about your personal life and how it is being forced into unnatural ways that you can do something about. For example, let grandmothers into your family life—and if you are one, it is normal to want to be with the grandchildren!

3. **Sunshine and Sunlight**

- It is normal to seek the sun. Try to get at least ten minutes exposure per day, in the middle of the day, without sunscreen. Just use common sense and, if you start to see reddening, that is the signal to stop and start again the next day.

- Sunlight (as opposed to sunshine) is also important. Get at least thirty minutes of full morning light (overcast is okay)—unlike indoor lighting, it is still bright enough to synchronize the body clock.

4. **Sleeping Patterns**

- Humans are designed to get some seven to eight hours of quality sleep per night.

- For a couple of hours after sunset, it is best to have lower levels of lighting—a flickering log fire is ideal! But in particular, avoid the bluish light given out by electronic devices.

- If you feel the need, a forty to fifty-minute siesta during the day is a normal, even healthful, thing to do.

CONCLUSION

In this section, we went over the ten factors of the Savanna Model eating pattern. We discussed various food groups: Grains, starchy and non-starchy plant foods, fruits, dairy products, meats, legumes, nuts, fats, sweeteners, salt, and beverages. Products in each food group were classified as "Green-Green" (safe to eat), "Amber" (tolerable), "Red" (avoid), or somewhere in between these categories, depending upon how well they fit into the Savanna Model criteria. To briefly summarize, grains, starches, dairy, legumes, sugar, and salt are to be avoided, while you may consume non-starchy vegetables in any amount you'd like. Fruits, some meats, nuts, and omega-3 fats are also safe to eat. Combining proper food choices and our natural lifestyle habits is the path to a long and healthful life.

If you have been eating a certain way for years, it can be difficult to change the type and quantity of food you consume. In the next chapter, we provide a more thorough guide to integrating this dietary plan into your daily life.

5.

Adopting the Paleo Feeding Pattern

O ur Pleistocene ancestors were not following any feeding strategies—they just followed their instincts. Their eating patterns would have changed from day to day according to the hazards of foraging. From season to season, their eating habits would have changed according to the availability of flora and fauna in the environment. Even so, the possible variations would have fallen within fairly strict limits.

Today, "what is there" is mostly artificial. The artful food manufacturers are masters at giving us taste without food value at all, and our instincts are readily duped by the divorce of taste from nutritional quality. The fluctuations of "what is there" fall within much wider limits. There is virtually no external discipline of what, and how much, we eat. So, we are obliged to adopt eating strategies.

Here, we look at ways for realizing the Savanna Model pattern. The objective is to give an example of the thought processes, the questioning, and the discipline that it is necessary to adopt it. Do not get fixated on the patterns described here. Within the boundaries of the Owner's Manual, there is a wide variety of ways you can organize your eating day. Use the examples given here to limber up the brain and begin working in a new paradigm. This is one aspect of the "Bond Effect," the art of putting the Savanna Model into practice.

EATING AT HOME

We favor eating at home whenever possible, because you have the most control over your food supply. Nevertheless, there will be times when you are obliged to eat away from home—in restaurants or at the homes of friends and family. Try to rid yourself of notions about which foods are to be eaten at which meals: For example, eggs are often thought of as being purely a breakfast food. In fact, you can eat them at any meal. The same goes for just about every dish: They can be eaten at any time of day. The following strategies are to help you make these changes to your way of eating. Refer to the Owner's Manual on page 53 for specific information on food groups.

Morning

Our Pleistocene ancestors would rouse themselves with the sunrise and gradually get organized for the day. By mid-morning, the first groups, having set off on foraging expeditions, would start to feed on what they found. We should be doing the same: Not rush into eating a heavy, early breakfast. Don't worry about hunger cravings—there won't be any unless your blood sugar is out of control (in which case, you need to be particularly careful to follow these recommendations). Suppress any prejudices you may have about the desirability of eating a "hearty" breakfast. Commercial interests have manipulated our ideas of breakfast, perhaps more than for any other meal. Just in the last fifty years, public relations consultants have manipulated the American public into accepting corn flakes and bacon as breakfast foods.

A common reaction when people hear about the Bond Effect for the first time is: "What on Earth can we now have for breakfast?" In fact, there are several options, many being a return to what our grandparents ate as children.

Breakfast Ideas

❑ **Strategy A—Eat Conforming Fruit.** A good time to eat fruit is a short time after waking up in the morning. Your stomach is empty (or should be). You can then eat small portions of conforming fruit all through the morning until lunch time. You will feel a little empty as the morning progresses, so you can then eat another portion of fruit. Eat until the feeling of emptiness is gone. You may have eaten a little or a lot, but it doesn't matter because nobody is counting. Remember that an important part of feeling satisfied has to do with putting our eating apparatus to work. That is, feeling the fruit on the lips and teeth, tearing a bite out, chomping it, grinding it in our mouths, and feeling the sensation against our tongues, gums, and mouth linings.

❑ **Strategy B—Eat Conforming Vegetables.** An alternative that is practiced in many parts of the world is to start the day with a vegetable stir-fry. This is what many societies in Asia do. Just take a bag of frozen, mixed vegetables and cook it in a saucepan using the "oil and water" method (see inset on page 88). Don't forget, you are using large quantities—at least 12 oz per person. If you like, you can add a few shrimp.

❑ **Strategy C—Eggs.** Omega-3-rich, free-range eggs any style are fine to start the day. Make a hearty vegetable-filled omelet or grill some tomatoes and mushrooms to go with the eggs. Don't forget that plant food should form the major part of the meal, and no backsliding—definitely no bread.

❑ **Strategy D—Salad.** The idea of eating salad for breakfast does indeed run counter to our Western cultural programming, but it is something that many societies do, notably in Africa. A copious mixed salad with some avocado, tuna

"Oil and Water" Cooking Method

Try this quick (five-minute) method of cooking vegetables. Put a quarter-inch of water into a saucepan with a sliced clove of garlic and a bay leaf (or a pinch of oregano). Add a tablespoon of canola oil. The boiling water forms an emulsion with the oil. Add vegetables (fresh or frozen). Heat moderately with the cover on, but stir frequently, too. The vegetables cook fast, partly by boiling and partly by steaming. At the end, when the vegetables are close to done, heat vigorously and stir continuously until all the water has gone. They will be a beautiful golden brown when the water has evaporated. Always use plenty of herbs. As many vegetables soak up oil, this method greatly reduces the quantity of oil absorbed.

flakes, or shrimp makes a great start to the day. Again, make it a large portion—at least one pound per person. It is not really so much: One large tomato, one cucumber, some onion, and some lettuce leaves make 9 oz of plant food. Round it off with 3 oz of canned tuna, and you have a hearty breakfast.

❏ **Strategy E—Old-Fashioned Haddock Breakfast.** This used to be a good standby in many parts of the English-speaking world. Many people are old enough to remember, perhaps, when their grandparents used to eat like this. They would lightly poach a piece of haddock (or kipper or any other appropriate fish) in simmering water for about five minutes. They would accompany it with lashings of sautéed onion, grilled tomatoes, and mushrooms.

❏ **Strategy F—The Savanna Model Continental Breakfast.** In Appendix B (Recipes), we suggest a sample of conforming dishes. They are all free of flour, dairy, butter, and sugar and are fully safe, even for diabetics. Some of these, such as almond flour bread, Paleo muesli, and marble ring cake, make excellent and tasty substitutes for croissants or Danish pastry.

Mid-Morning

Depending on how you started the day, you can snack on an avocado, a handful of raw unsalted nuts, or a big bowl of homemade vegetable soup. Select vegetables from Food Group 3 (Non-starchy Vegetables). Get used to making extra large quantities of everything and make sure that the fridge or freezer has a ready supply of easily accessed foods.

Lunch Time

A suitable choice for lunch is a mixed salad, and an appropriate quantity might be 12 oz. Weigh foods until you are used to estimating the quantities by eye—it's larger than you are used to. Get in the habit of thinking that a salad is often in two parts: The salad vegetables, comprised uniquely of foods from Food

Group 3 (Non-starchy Vegetables), and some additions of protein-rich foods from Food Group 6 (Meat, Poultry, Eggs, and Fish). You can add tuna or chicken breast, for example, to the salad or eat as a side dish. Use a simple homemade vinaigrette of mustard, olive oil, lemon juice, and vinegar.

Preferably, eat the salad before the side dish, because your appetite will be more readily satisfied by the bulkiest part of the meal. Eating the low-density plant food takes time. This gives time for the complex signaling from stomach to brain to catch up and tell you to feel satisfied.

Afternoon Snacks

Through the afternoon, you may begin to feel hungry. Keep ready prepared in your fridge some raw broccoli, cauliflower, and baby carrots, and also have some containers of preservative-free dips, such as guacamole. Get used to taking your fuel with you when you are away from home for several hours. Above all, overcome any inhibitions you may have about pulling it out and eating it when the occasion calls.

Dinner Time

Dinner involves the same decision-making process as at lunch time. This time you decide to do some cooking. Maybe 12 oz per person of stir-fried vegetables accompanied by two eggs, any style. Or a grilled trout with a head of steamed broccoli. It's as easy as that.

The stir-fry can be ready frozen; season with garlic, lemon juice, and herbs. Note that we are escaping the tyranny of the "starter, main course, and dessert" regimen. Instead, it's just the one course. As ever, try to eat the vegetables before anything else. A glass of dry wine is okay, too.

See the recipes in Appendix B for ideas about vegetable, poultry, seafood, and meat dishes.

Bedtime (Supper)

For a snack before bedtime, if there has been a sufficient gap after the last meal, eat a low-glycemic fruit (as much as you like). If not, try 1 oz of nuts. Avoid bad carbohydrates this late in the day—they provoke a hormonal reaction that disturbs sleep and interferes with the body's nighttime repair processes. If you fancy it, have a mug of cocoa or about .75 oz of dark chocolate (made up of at least 75 percent cocoa solids).

EATING AWAY FROM HOME

It is one thing to be organized at home for eating in accordance with the Savanna Model, but it is quite another matter when away from home. However, by planning ahead, being assertive, and being prepared, it is quite possible to stay close to the ideal regimen.

Restaurants

In reasonable-quality restaurants, it is relatively simple to find items on the menu that can form the basis of a meal. I say "form the basis" because you will still have to ask questions and request changes: "What exactly does the salad have in it? I don't want any croutons, pasta, rice, or fruit." (Remember that fruit, even conforming fruit, should not be eaten with other food groups.) So it goes, until you have selected the starter, main course, and dessert.

Pay close attention to the vegetables that accompany the main course and refuse potatoes (including French fries) and rice, which restaurants often offer as "vegetables." If green beans, broccoli, spinach, or any other green vegetable is available, ask for double portions. Firmly wave away the bread basket and leave any sweet corn on the plate. Most of the desserts will be off-limits. When you have finished such a meal, you can congratulate yourself—you have eaten healthily and within the margins of tolerance.

Eating in fast-food restaurants is a little harder. Find a salad, if you can; discard the packet of salad dressing, unless it is simple oil and vinegar. Consider carrying a bottle of your own vinaigrette. Or eat the all-day breakfast: Eggs with tomatoes and mushrooms (without bread or roll) are acceptable, but avoid the bacon, sausage, hash browns, toast, waffles, syrup, and muffins. It is not ideal to eat the processed meat in fast-food restaurants, but if you must, order the burger (no cheese) or grilled chicken sandwich and throw away the bun.

Many fast-food restaurants have salad bars. This is good news and, with care, one can eat reasonably correctly. They do tend to drench the salads in sweetened dressings. Often they mix in fruit or combine starches and proteins. Be selective: Pick out and put aside the offending ingredients. Be suspicious of all salad dressings—the manufacturers invariably make them with low-quality ingredients, fillers, and sugars. Do the best you can.

Dinner Parties

In some ways, a dinner party is the hardest situation to manage. You don't want to put your hosts under pressure, and you want to be invited another day. If you know your hosts well, it is all right to call in advance and mention that you have special dietary requirements. Say that you prefer fish over red meat or that you don't like to eat fruit after a meal. Mention that you like green salads and lots of green vegetables. Then, dig into your meal and enjoy it for what it is. You will certainly have to compromise, but if your basic eating habits are natural and healthy, the occasional lapse is not going to be the end of the world.

If you don't know your hosts well, or the dinner party has a set menu, then it is best to act defensively. Before setting off, eat a light meal of conforming plant food (salad, vegetables, nuts, and so on). Then, when you get to your dinner, eat lightly. The "allergy excuse" is always accepted if you want to leave a significant portion on your plate. People also understand if you are watching your waistline and don't want to eat much of the dessert. You can escape from this challenge in pretty good order.

PREPARING AND COOKING FOOD

In our African Pleistocene past, our ancestors did indeed have fire, but they had no way to boil water. They generally ate plant food raw, although they often roasted tubers and sometimes roasted nuts and other materials. Animal matter, according to convenience, type, and body part, was eaten raw or roasted. Eggs were also eaten raw. These are generalities, but we can combine this with what we know about how cooking affects nutrition.

In the Savanna Model, the emphasis is on keeping meals simple and eating raw when you can and cooking when you must. Vegetables should be used as fresh as possible. Store them in a cool, airy place like the vegetable rack of the refrigerator. Most vegetables can (and should) be eaten raw. Frozen vegetables are acceptable. Canned vegetables are acceptable in controlled situations where the convenience outweighs the nutritional drawbacks. Canned tomatoes, for example, are still quite wholesome and are useful in "quick-fix" dishes. Think big for your utensils. The food quantities are at least double what you are used to. Get a large salad bowl, frying pan, and saucepan.

With regard to plant food, it is always best to eat it as soon as possible after harvesting and to eat it raw. That is why we put the emphasis on the consumption of salads and for them to be as fresh as possible. Be imaginative—many vegetables can form part of a mixed salad, including chopped broccoli, cauliflower, cabbage, zucchini, and leeks. With that big salad in place in your diet, it is acceptable to consume cooked vegetables, too. However, the process should be quick to avoid leaching of nutrients. Always use the minimum amount of cooking possible so that the vegetable is still "al dente," that is, cooked to keep its crunchy texture.

The best method for cooking vegetables is steaming or blanching. For example, you can cook broccoli florets in boiling water for three minutes, which will minimize nutrient loss. Microwave steaming is acceptable, although it is more aggressive on nutrient loss. Light stir-frying is also an acceptable cooking method. Stir-frying in the traditional Chinese method uses no oil, just a couple of teaspoons of water. Steaming, steam microwaving, and blanching are all good ways to cook vegetables. Avoid lengthy boiling, deep-frying, and roasting.

Frozen, chopped vegetables are a good standby. They can be stir-fried, just as they come, in their own juices. No need to use a wok—just heat rapidly and stir constantly for five to six minutes in a large saucepan. Always use plenty of herbs. The basic stir-fry herb mixture contains oregano, crushed bay leaves, basil, and thyme. You can make up your own mix using equal parts of these herbs, or find a product that conforms closely to this recipe. Use the "oil and water" cooking method described on page 88.

Foods of animal origin can be cooked. In general terms, there are few nutrients that might be destroyed by heating. Even oily fish keep their good omega-3 oils intact after baking, grilling, or barbecuing. One of the reasons we recommend avoiding red meats is not only their high content of bad fats, but also the fact that the fat oxidizes under high heat. Oxidized fat is a biochemical disaster for health. Meat, poultry, eggs, and fish (Food Group 6) can be cooked using the most appropriate method: Microwaving, steaming, grilling, baking, or sautéing. Avoid deep-frying. If using oil, just use a light coating of olive oil.

You do not need to make fancy dishes every day. In fact, we encourage you to eat simply. Nevertheless, there are many occasions when such dishes are appreciated, particularly for dinner parties and even as useful snacks at home, school, or work.

Preserved Foods

"Fresh is best" is a familiar slogan and it is good for us, too. However, that is not always possible, so how do we prioritize? Broadly speaking, the "least bad" alternative to fresh plant food is frozen. Frozen plant foods, such as cauliflower, spinach, and chopped onion, have been quickly prepared in the field, and then blanched and frozen nearby. Blanching is designed to destroy certain enzymes that cause discoloration, softening, and bruising. It is likely that these are background micronutrients that are useful to the human body and become lost in the blanching process. So, here we make a compromise: In the absence of an alternative, freezing is the least of all evils.

The other methods of preserving plant food are to be avoided: Freeze-dried (packet soups), canned (peas, green beans), pickled in salt (gherkins), syruped (fruit jams and jellies), and fermented (sauerkraut). That is not to say you can never eat these things, just do not think that they are proper food. Foods pickled in vinegar (such as onions) have lost many nutrients, but at least the pickling does not add undesirable chemicals.

With regard to animal matter, many methods of conservation are acceptable. Canned oily fish (such as sardines) are, in nutritional terms, just as good as fresh. Just choose the versions that are preserved in olive oil, canola oil, or unsalted water. Smoked salmon or kipper are good, although watch out for high salt content. Frozen poultry, fish, seafood, and exotic meats are fine too. Pickled fish (like herring) are acceptable, but be watchful of the salt and sugar content. Cured meats (such as bacon, ham, sausage, and bologna) are to be avoided simply because they contain high levels of fat, bad fats, salt, and sulfites. They are often heavily processed, as well (see "Processed and Manufactured Foods" below).

Processed and Manufactured Foods

Eat food that is as minimally processed as possible. As a rough guide, if a product is sold with an ingredients label, then it is processed and you should thoroughly vet it. Processing destroys fibers and leaches out valuable micronutrients. Processing increases the glycemic index and almost always means the addition of unwanted, useless, and sometimes harmful compounds—artificial coloring, artificial flavoring, preservatives, emulsifiers, stabilizers, and fungicides (like sodium propionate). Harmful ingredients like sugars, salt, trans fats, and hydrogenated fat are frequently added. The manufacturers adulterate and thin down their products with a variety of junk fillers like whey, modified starch, and unbleached wheat flour.

Government authorities allow meat packers to inject saltwater into products like ham, bacon, and chicken breasts.[1] You do not need the salt and you might object to paying up to 25 percent of the price just for water. Take your fine reading glasses with you to the supermarket (even health food stores are not necessarily safe) and read the ingredient labels. Avoid the bad carbohydrates, shy away from products that have lengthy ingredient lists, and avoid oils and fat additives, particularly animal fats and hydrogenated fats.

Genetically Modified Organisms (GMOs)

Biotechnology companies produce genetically modified plants for many reasons, but rarely to increase nutrition. Governments and the industry hasten to reassure the public that genetically modified organisms (GMOs) are safe, but that is not the point. Volcanic ash might be safe to eat, but is it food? Already our current food supply is too far removed from the Savanna Model. After all, we are organic creatures that have grown up in harmony with a particular pattern of naturally occurring vegetation and fauna.

Most Americans do not realize how much of their food supply—some 75 percent of it—is infiltrated by GMOs, particularly anything containing tomato, soy, and corn (maize).[2] In America, no authority requires the presence of these GMOs to be labeled.[3] In contrast, the European Union (EU) requires all foodstuffs containing GMOs to be so labeled.[4] However, all is not lost for Americans. After an outcry from consumers, the U.S. Department of Agriculture (USDA) backtracked and agreed that the "organic" label could not be applied to genetically modified foods.[5]

As things stand, genetically modified food is probably "safe" and nutritionally similar to plants produced by regular intensive farming, but no one knows for sure. Nevertheless, avoid GMOs where you can and consume them when you must. There is also a stronger reason to avoid GMOs: The ethical one of combating the agro-industry mentality that recklessly dumps fake food onto our plates.

Organic Foods

Organic plant food is usually much richer in micronutrients than food from intensively farmed (conventional) plants.[6] It is less likely to contain pesticides and other chemicals. Moreover, its production methods are kinder to the landscape and its animal husbandry practices are usually more caring. Organic foods of the Savanna Model will always be best. But is "organic" the first priority? Not necessarily. One of the greatest dietary errors in the West is the low consumption of plant food. The adverse health consequences are grave and measurable; the consequences of eating agro-industrial versions rather than organic are smaller. Therefore, the highest priority is to eat more Savanna Model food from whatever source. Eating organic is a second order of priority.

The designation "organic" does not turn a bad food into a good one. Organic sugar, organic milk, organic butter, and organic pork are all just as bad as the regular sort. Does a cigarette smoker worry if his tobacco is organic? Of course not—the main problem is the tobacco itself.

So, choose organic when you can; otherwise, select conventionally produced foods when you must. For this to happen, your attitudes will have to change. In particular, be prepared to pay a little more. Also, be prepared for produce that is more misshapen, bruised, and discolored—buy organic and shun the Technicolor perfection of supermarket produce. You will be rewarded by glorious, rich flavors and the comfort of knowing that you are nourishing your body with genuine nutrients.

ADOPTING THE SAVANNA MODEL IN THREE STAGES

When you start to eat naturally, you are making major changes in the structure of how and what you eat. These changes have repercussions and may be uncomfortable during the transition phase. That is why it is wise to introduce the changes gradually.

Put in place the new, healthy eating habits of the Savanna Model in Stage 1 and then move on to the other stages. Step by step, you will gradually modify your habits in the right direction, substituting healthy choices for your current unhealthy ones. Over the course of the three stages, you will slowly wean yourself from the foods that are not good for you and start to incorporate more and more of the Savanna Model.

Take it at a pace that is comfortable for you. You can even decide to stop at some intermediate stage. Each stage is a summary of the more detailed advice already given in the book. If in doubt, refer back to the earlier chapters. For each stage, there follows examples of foodstuffs in the various categories used in the Owner's Manual (refer back to page 53).

Earlier in this chapter, we gave an example of how we might eat during the day. Typically, we would eat less at a time but more often. Some might be light meals taken at regular mealtimes like lunch or dinner; others are light meals taken between them, like afternoon tea and supper. In the following segment, we talk about these eating occasions as "sessions." We also refer to eating a certain number of servings of each food group. For specific measurements of "one serving," please see the "Serving Sizes" inset on page 95.

Serving Sizes

In the following sections, we refer to eating a certain number of servings of each food group per day or per week. The serving sizes we recommend are the same as those of the American Heart Association (AHA):[7]

■ **Food Group 1—Grains and Seeds:** Examples of one serving include one slice of bread; half a bagel; 2 tablespoons (1 oz) dry cereal; $1/2$ cup cooked rice, pasta, or cereal; 2 tablespoons seeds.

■ **Food Groups 2 and 3—Starchy and Non-starchy Vegetables:** Examples of one serving include 1 cup raw, leafy vegetables; $1/2$ cup cut up raw or cooked vegetables; $1/2$ cup of vegetable juice.

■ **Food Group 4—Fruits:** Examples of one serving include 1 medium (baseball-sized) fruit; $1/4$ cup dried fruit; $1/2$ cup frozen, fresh, or canned fruit; $1/2$ cup fruit juice.

■ **Food Group 5—Dairy and Cheese:** Examples of one serving include 1 cup milk; 1 cup yogurt; 3 tablespoons ($11/2$ oz) cheese; $1/2$ cup ice cream.

■ **Food Group 6—Meat, Poultry, Eggs, Fish:** Examples of one serving include 3 oz (size of a deck of cards) cooked meat or poultry; 3 oz grilled fish; 1 egg.

■ **Food Group 7—Legumes:** Examples of one serving include $1/2$ cup dry beans, peas, etc; 2 tablespoons peanut butter.

■ **Food Group 8—Nuts:** Examples of one serving include $1/3$ cup nuts; 2 tablespoons almond, cashew, etc. butter (*not* peanut butter).

■ **Food Group 9—Fats and Oils:** Examples of one serving include 1 teaspoon margarine; 1 tablespoon mayonnaise or spread; 1 teaspoon canola, vegetable, olive, fish, coconut, etc. oil.

■ **Food Group 10—Sugars:** Examples of one serving include 1 tablespoon sugar, honey, sugar substitute, jelly, or jam; $1/2$ cup sorbet.

■ **Food Group 11—Salt and Sodium:** The AHA does not have serving sizes listed for salt and sodium, but recommends that you eat no more than 2,300 mg (1 teaspoon table salt) per day.[8] Of course, in the Owner's Manual, I recommended you eat even less—as little as possible. Make sure you balance your sodium intake with your potassium intake.

■ **Food Group 12—Beverages:** The recommended serving sizes of beverages depends on what sort of beverage it is. One half-cup is one serving of fruit or vegetable juice. One cup is one serving of water, milk, or nut milk.

For most foods not specified above, one serving size is generally 3 oz—about the size of a small fist or a deck of cards. A serving of most fatty, sugary, or salty foods should be about 1 tablespoon.

Stage 1

This stage is the most important—you have opened the portal to a new world, one that will change your life. Most of the changes are not difficult: Much of it is the simple exchange of one food for an equal substitute. Other changes have to do with the order in which foods are eaten. None of it demands a lot of willpower.

Cooking and Food Preparation

- Avoid deep-frying.

- Reduce consumption of processed foods, fast foods, ready meals, etc., to no more than one serving per day.

Dietary Tips

- Eat fruit on an empty stomach.

- Avoid protein/starch combinations.

Accumulation of Lapses

Across all food groups together, limit your servings of Red, Red-Amber, and Amber foods in the following way.

- "Red" foods—limit to no more than four per day.

- "Red-Amber" foods—limit to no more than six per day.

- "Amber" foods—limit to no more than eight per day.

STAGE 1
FOOD GROUP 1   GRAINS
Have one day per week bread-free.
Have three days per week free of pizza, breakfast cereals, and pasta.
FOOD GROUP 2   STARCHY VEGETABLES
Restrict French fries to no more than three servings per week.
Have one day per week free of "Red" foods. On the other days, limit "Red" foods to one serving per day.
Have one day per week free of "Amber-Red" foods. On the other days, limit "Amber-Red" foods to two servings per day.
FOOD GROUP 3   NON-STARCHY VEGETABLES
Eat at least a half-pound of mixed salad per day, consisting of "Green-Green" and "Green" foods.
Eat at least a half-pound of cooked vegetables per day, consisting of "Green-Green" and "Green" foods.

STAGE 1 *continued*

FOOD GROUP 4   FRUIT

Eat at least one piece (serving) of fruit per day.

Focus on "Green" and "Green-Amber" fruits.

Avoid "Amber-Red" fruits.

Eat no more than one serving of "Amber" fruit per session.

Eat no more than three servings of fruit per session.

FOOD GROUP 5   DAIRY

Replace whole milk with skim.

Drink no more than one cup of milk per day.

Limit ice cream to three servings per week.

Limit cheese to one serving per day.

FOOD GROUP 6   MEAT, POULTRY, EGGS, AND FISH

Use only omega-3-rich, free-range eggs.

Consume at least three servings a week of "Green-Green" foods.

Limit "Red," "Amber-Red," and "Amber" foods to no more than three servings per week.

Reduce total food group servings per day to two.

FOOD GROUP 7   LEGUMES

Reduce consumption of "Red" foods to no more than three servings per week.

Reduce consumption of "Amber-Red" foods to no more than seven servings per week.

FOOD GROUP 8   NUTS

Consume at least three servings each of "Green-Green" and "Green" foods per week.

Restrict total food group servings per day to two.

Restrict total food group servings per session to one.

FOOD GROUP 9   FATS AND OILS

Use one tablespoon of "Green-Green" oils at least three times a week.

Limit "Amber-Red" fats and oils to five tablespoons per week.

Avoid "Red" fats and oils.

Replace butter and margarine with "Green" spreads.

Replace cream with almond or coconut cream.

Restrict total servings of this food group to five tablespoons per day.

STAGE 1 *continued*

FOOD GROUP 10   SUGARS AND SWEETENERS

Replace "Red" table sugar with "Green-Amber" sugars.

Limit intake of "Red" sweeteners to 2 oz per day.

Avoid overdosing on fructose, agave syrup, and sugar replacements.

Limit intake of "Green-Amber" sweeteners to 1 $1/_2$ oz per day.

Limit intake of "Green" sweeteners to 1 oz per session.

FOOD GROUP 11   SALT AND SODIUM

Replace "Red" seasonings with "Amber" (or better) seasonings.

FOOD GROUP 12   BEVERAGES

Replace regular colas and soft drinks with "diet" versions.

Eliminate sweetened fruit juices.

Focus on "Green" and "Green-Amber" beverages.

Reduce consumption of "Amber" beverages to five or less servings (12 oz mug or can) per day.

Reduce consumption of "Amber-Red" beverages to two or less servings (12 oz mug or can) per day.

Reduce consumption of "Red" beverages to one serving (12 oz mug or can) per day.

Stage 2

In this stage, we turn the screw a little tighter, but when you have mastered it, you will have escaped the gravity of your old earth-bound ways. You are "over the hump" and are already fueling your body in ways that has learned to recognize and respond to.

Cooking and Food Preparation

- Avoid deep-frying.
- Reduce boiling and roasting; prefer stir-frying, steaming, and microwave steaming.
- Reduce consumption of processed foods to no more than three servings per week.
- Keep meals simple.
- Eat little but often.
- Spend at least thirty minutes, once per day, feeling slightly hungry.

Dietary Tips

- Eat fruit on its own (i.e., do not include it in a meal with other foods).
- Avoid protein/starch combinations.

Accumulation of Lapses

Across all food groups together, limit your servings of Red, Red-Amber, and Amber foods in the following way.

- "Red" foods—limit to no more than one serving per day.
- "Amber-Red" foods—limit to no more than two servings per day.
- "Amber" foods—limit to no more than three servings per day.

STAGE 2

FOOD GROUP 1   GRAINS

Have four days per week free of "Red" foods. On other days, limit "Red" foods to one serving per day.

Have three days per week free of "Amber-Red" foods. On other days, limit "Amber-Red" foods to one serving per day.

FOOD GROUP 2   STARCHY VEGETABLES

Eliminate French fries.

Have four days per week free of "Red" foods. On other days, limit "Red" foods to one serving per day.

Have three days per week free of "Amber-Red" foods. On other days, limit "Amber-Red" foods to one serving per day.

FOOD GROUP 3   NON-STARCHY VEGETABLES

Eat at least three servings per week of "Green-Green" foods.

Eat at least $1^1/_2$ lbs of salads and vegetables per day, "Green-Green" and "Green."

FOOD GROUP 4   FRUIT

Eat at least three servings of fruit per day, focusing on "Green" and "Green-Amber" fruits.

Avoid "Amber-Red" fruits.

Restrict consumption of "Amber" fruits to one serving per session.

Restrict consumption of total fruits to three servings per session.

FOOD GROUP 5   DAIRY

Replace cow's milk with unsweetened almond milk.

Eliminate "Red" foods.

Limit consumption of cheese to 3 oz or less, three times a week.

STAGE 2 *continued*

FOOD GROUP 6   MEAT, POULTRY, EGGS, AND FISH

Preferably consume two servings per day of "Green-Green" and/or "Green" foods.

Limit consumption of "Amber" foods to one serving a week.

Limit consumption of "Amber-Red" foods to one serving a month.

Eliminate "Red" foods.

Use only omega-3-rich, free-range hen's eggs.

Restrict total of food group servings per session to one.

Restrict total of food group servings per day to two.

FOOD GROUP 7   LEGUMES

Eliminate "Red" foods.

Consume no more than one serving per week of "Red-Amber" foods.

FOOD GROUP 8   NUTS

Consume at least three servings per week of "Green" foods.

Consume at least five servings per week of "Green-Green" foods.

Restrict total food group servings per session to one.

Restrict total food group servings per day to two.

FOOD GROUP 9   FATS AND OILS

Use one tablespoon of "Green-Green" oil at least seven times a week.

Avoid all "Amber-Red" and "Red" fats.

Replace butter and margarine with "Green" spreads.

Replace cream with almond or coconut cream.

Restrict total food group servings per day to five tablespoons.

FOOD GROUP 10   SUGARS AND SWEETENERS

Avoid all "Red" sweeteners; replace with "Green-Amber."

Limit consumption of "Green-Amber" foods to 1 oz per day.

Limit consumption of "Green" foods to 1 oz per session.

FOOD GROUP 11   SALT AND SODIUM

Avoid all "Red" and "Amber-Red" seasonings. Replace with "Amber" or better seasonings.

Eliminate added salt in cooking; replace with herbs and flavoring like lemon juice.

STAGE 2 *continued*
FOOD GROUP 12   BEVERAGES
Focus on "Green" and "Green-Amber" beverages. Restrict consumption of freshly-pressed fruit juices to three servings per week. Consume no more than three 12 oz servings of "Amber" beverages per week. Consume no more than two 12 oz servings of "Amber-Red" beverages per week. Eliminate sweetened fruit juices.

Stage 3

By the time you have completed this stage, you will be in conformity with the Savanna Model and you will be feeding your body in its comfort zone. You will discover the good things that happen when your biochemistry and digestive system are functioning as nature intended. Fighting a life-threatening degenerative disease? Then this stage is for you. Get to the center of the comfort zone, where your body is not just coping, it is positively rejoicing with its newfound ability to hum along like a perfectly adjusted machine.

Cooking and Food Preparation

- Reduce consumption of processed foods to no more than three servings per month.
- Prefer organic foods wherever available.
- Avoid deep-frying; reduce boiling and roasting; prefer stir-frying, steaming, and microwave steaming.
- Keep meals simple.
- Eat little but often.
- Spend at least thirty minutes, three times per day, feeling slightly hungry.

Dietary Tips

- Eat fruit on its own.
- Avoid protein/starch combinations.

Accumulation of Lapses

Across all food groups together, limit your servings of Red, Amber-Red, and Amber foods in the following way.

- "Red" foods—limit to no more than one per week.
- "Amber-Red" foods—limit to no more than two per week.
- "Amber" foods—limit to no more than three per week.

STAGE 3

FOOD GROUP 1   GRAINS

Eliminate all "Red" and "Amber-Red" products.

FOOD GROUP 2   STARCHY VEGETABLES

Eliminate all "Red" and "Amber-Red" foods.

Limit consumption of "Amber" foods to three servings per week, and no more than one serving per day.

FOOD GROUP 3   NON-STARCHY VEGETABLES

Eat at least 2 3/4 lbs of mixed salad and vegetables per day, consisting of "Green-Green" and "Green" foods. Of these, at least 3/4 lb should be mixed salad. Also include at least 5 cups of "Green-Green" leafy vegetables or 2 1/2 cups of other vegetables per week.

Limit consumption of "Amber" foods to five servings per week and no more than one serving per day.

Limit consumption of "Amber-Red" foods to one serving a week.

FOOD GROUP 4   FRUITS

Eat at least six pieces (servings) of fruit per day, focusing on "Green" and "Green-Amber" fruits.

Restrict total of "Amber" fruits per session to one serving.

Eliminate "Amber-Red" fruits.

Restrict total fruits consumption per session to three servings.

FOOD GROUP 5   DAIRY

Eliminate "Red" and "Amber-Red" foods.

FOOD GROUP 6   MEAT, POULTRY, EGGS, AND FISH

Preferably consume two servings a day of "Green-Green" foods. If unavailable, you can consume two servings a day of "Green" foods.

Limit consumption of "Amber" foods to one serving a month.

Eliminate "Red" and "Amber-Red" foods.

Use only omega-3-rich, free-range, organic hen's eggs.

Restrict total food group servings per session to one.

Restrict total food group servings per day to two.

FOOD GROUP 7   LEGUMES

Eliminate "Red" and "Amber-Red" foods.

STAGE 3 *continued*

FOOD GROUP 8 NUTS

Consume at least three servings of "Green" foods per week.
Consume at least seven servings of "Green-Green" foods per week.
Restrict total nuts servings per session to one.
Restrict total nuts servings per day to two.

FOOD GROUP 9 FATS AND OILS

Use 1 tablespoons of "Green-Green" oil at least seven times a week.
Avoid all "Amber-Red" and "Red" fats and oils.
Replace butter and margarine with "Green" spreads.
Replace cream with almond or coconut cream.
Restrict total fats and oils consumption to 5 tablespoons (80 ml) per day.

FOOD GROUP 10 SUGARS AND SWEETENERS

Avoid all "Red" sugars and sweeteners.
Limit consumption of "Amber" foods to 2 oz (60 grams) per week.
Limit intake of "Green-Amber" foods to 1 oz (30 mg) per day.
Limit intake of "Green" foods to 1 oz (30 mg) per session.

FOOD GROUP 11 SALT AND SODIUM

Avoid all "Red," "Amber-Red," and "Amber" seasonings.
When cooking and eating, use herbs and flavorings like lemon juice.

FOOD GROUP 12 BEVERAGES

Focus on "Green" and "Green-Amber" beverages.
Avoid all "Red," "Amber-Red," and "Amber" beverages.

WHAT TO EXPECT AS YOU CHANGE YOUR DIET

As you enter each subsequent stage of the Savanna Model eating pattern, your digestive system may be in a state of shock, at least temporarily. If you have been following a Western diet for years, you have, unwittingly, been abusing and mistreating your digestive system. Many of its functions will have shut down. Your new way of eating will bring some immediate benefits: For example, elimination of bad food combining will dramatically reduce digestive problems. The increase in soluble fiber from fruits and vegetables will force lazy and atrophied intestinal muscles to limber up and become operational again. But be prepared for bouts of diarrhea or constipation for several weeks—this is normal during the transition period.

You will also start to lose excess fat from your body—that is the good news. However, as the glucagon machinery swings into action, fat will dissolve into your bloodstream, delivering its cargo of unpleasant chemicals. While the body eliminates them, you may suffer discomfort from their presence in the blood. Be prepared for symptoms, such as increased allergy activity, headaches, and feeling "one degree under," during the transition period.

Food is a potent factor for modifying the hormones in the body. As you shift the emphasis on what you eat, particularly from "bad" carbohydrates to "good" carbohydrates, you will be modifying your hormonal balance. During the transition period, you may feel the effects: Mood swings, sugar cravings, and headaches, for example. This is normal.

Once you have restructured your way of eating, you will find that bowel movements will occur once or twice a day. They are soft and easy to expel, do not have a noxious odor, and are copious in quantity. Food will have a rapid transit time through the digestive tract. When you get to this point, you will know for sure that you are eating correctly. Rejoice at the wholesome feeling of health and tone in your intestines. The friendly flora and fauna will flourish, providing most of the bulk in the feces. Instead of having a clogged-up sewer system for a gut, your digestive system nurtures a health-giving, symbiotic biomass.

When you eat in accordance with the Savanna Model, mouth hygiene is also vastly improved. The mechanical action of chewing a high volume of raw vegetable matter stimulates and hardens (keratinizes) the gums. Saliva quality is also improved; most people on a Western diet have a deregulated saliva composition. The saliva should contain a balanced cocktail of enzymes and antibacterial agents. Once you are eating in accordance with the Savanna Model, the saliva finds its equilibrium and fulfills a major role: Keeping the mouth microbiome wholesome and sweet-smelling. If you have poor tooth and gum health, do the best you can to get it fixed: Often, people are pushed into poor food choices just because they cannot chew the right foods comfortably.

HOW DOES THE SAVANNA MODEL APPLY TO ME?

The Savanna Model applies to everybody, but here we look at the specific implications for various groups, including babies and toddlers, children and adolescents, pregnant and nursing women, the elderly, and others. Each of these groups is in a different stage of development in life, and thus their eating patterns need to be tailored to their bodies' capabilities.

Babies and Toddlers

Up to the age of about four years, human babies are "lactivores," or milk drinkers. Nature designed them to nourish themselves on human breast milk. In primitive societies, babies are not fully weaned until they are about four years old, although solid foods, sometimes partially pre-masticated by their mothers, are introduced slowly from about twelve months of age. That is the ideal, but what to do in the modern world? Mercifully, the breastfeeding movement has made this practice not only acceptable, but also practical. Today, mothers can give breast to their child in public places, something unthinkable as recently as the 1960s. The vast majority of mothers in the industrialized world, neverthe-less, find it hard to breastfeed after about twelve months, let alone to pre-masti-cate pap for a two-year-old.

Fortunately, the companies that make formula milk are getting very good at making a product that imitates human milk as closely as possible. As a reminder, you have to avoid soy-based formula milks. Most countries ban them because their anti-nutrients harm babies' health, but they are still widely avail-able in the U.S.[9] In other respects, formula milks have come a long way in the last fifty years: No more cow's milk allergens, a healthier ratio of fats to proteins, and a much better composition of vitamins, minerals, and essential fatty acids. They now have products that mimic the fact that the composition of mother's milk changes as the baby gets older. For example, in the first weeks of life, a baby's biochemistry cannot use the essential fatty acids linoleic acid and alpha-linolenic acid. During this time, the mother's milk (and now specialized formula milks) contain compounds that compensate for this.

However, mother's milk contains antibodies and other compounds that protect the baby from disease early in life; formula milk cannot provide these. So, breastfeed if you can and for as long as you can, then move onto, and sup-plement with, the best formula milk you can find.

What about solid foods? The first principle is to follow the Savanna Model. The more the baby eats in accordance with the general principles formulated in this book, the better. Second, since people like to eat what they have always eaten, the best start in life for your baby is to give him or her the taste for healthy foods. When they are used to eating healthy foods at this stage, that liking will stay with them for life.

The first good habit to instill is the eating of plant food. No need to make special arrangements: Just take what you, as a Bond Effect practitioner, eat every day and reduce it down to a form appropriate to the child's stage of develop-ment. Today's food blenders, while not replicating the saliva input, are a reason-able substitute for the masticating jaws of the mother.

The next solid to be introduced should be fruit. However, take the precau-tions that we make for everybody: Focus on the lower-sugar, lower-glycemic fruits (the "Green" category). Do not give too much at one time and give it on an empty stomach; no point in making your baby's life a misery by bad food combining. Give fruits to your baby every day.

What about animal matter? Of course, many people bring up their children successfully as vegetarians. However, staying with the Savanna Model, fish and fowl are fine. Free-range, omega-3-rich eggs are always good in any quantity. Just remember, you don't have to give your child anything that, as a Bond Effect practitioner, you would not eat yourself.

In addition, a baby has a bigger need for the essential fatty acids (in a ratio of 1:1 for omega-3s and omega-6s) than an adult. There are at least two other fatty acids that their immature bodies are not capable of manufacturing for themselves: DHA (docosahexaenoic acid) and ARA (arachidonic acid). However, don't worry about them too much, because the infant fed in accordance with the Savanna Model will not be deficient in either DHA or ARA.

There will certainly be times when it is just not possible to prepare your own baby food. What about the commercially available products? Here, again, food manufacturers have gotten a lot more clever about formulating reasonably healthy substitutes. When you go shopping, the same rules apply—take your reading glasses and scrutinize the ingredient labels. Don't be misled by the attractive marketing labels proclaiming "healthy," "low-fat," "no artificial additives," etc. The food manufacturers always put the advantages of their product in large lettering, while the truth is grudgingly portrayed in small print in a corner of the label. This time, you are reading the ingredient list for a dependent baby, so be conscientious. Don't buy anything that contains ingredients that you would not want for yourself: Salt, sugar, glucose syrup, vegetable oil, fat, starch, and so on.

Finally, if your infant is not drinking mother's milk or formula milk, then the only other beverage he or she should have is plain water. Will any kind of water do? Tap water, unjustly, is much maligned and is quite safe to use when boiled. For all young babies, you should boil the water anyway. For the cautious, by all means buy bottled water. Avoid the high-sodium brands and varieties that are flavored with sugars. Distilled water is the safest. Juiced non-starchy vegetables are fine, but avoid carrot juice and fruit juices—they give a sugar rush and help rot teeth. As for packaged drinks, be ultra-suspicious. Read the fine print, as they are almost always loaded with sugar and other harmful substances. Don't even think of giving your child colas and other carbonated drinks. Get your child to accept water as the normal thirst-quencher.

Don't forget, this is one phase in your child's life when he or she is most open to influence from adults. It is now that you have to indoctrinate good consumption reflexes. This is not the time to introduce your child to pizzas, hamburgers, take-out chicken, or hot dogs. Even less is it the time to introduce your child to candies, cookies, ice cream, and confectionary. If you can get him or her through this phase without ever having tasted them, then you are well on the way to insulating your child from addiction later on.

Many adult health problems are established in these formative years. Perhaps the most significant is obesity. If your baby is allowed to get overweight, then the chances are that he will be overweight, or even obese, for the rest of his life. Worse, if your baby is overweight, he or she is already laying down plaque in the arteries and storing up a mid-life heart attack, as well as laying the foundations for cancer, arthritis, and a host of degenerative diseases.

Children/Adolescents

The special needs of children and adolescents are often exaggerated. They will be eating a lot for their size, but they do not need any particular divergence from the Savanna Model. By far the greatest problem is to stop them from eating harmful foods. It is too much to expect that you can hold back the floodwaters of the junk food society. Accept with good grace that your child will eat junk food from time to time, but don't be defeatist. Make sure that at home, he or she is following the Savanna Model. If that is assured, then your child will survive the storms of junk food relatively unscathed.

Avoid using junk food as a treat, much less as a reward. Rather, you need to indoctrinate children with the idea that junk food is shoddy, tacky, malignant, even hazardous, toxic, and poisonous. Children will accept that they are different from their peers if you present it as their particular belief system. You need to give them the arguments and words to use when well-meaning friends and relatives question their eating habits. Let them understand that they are eating in a way that avoids the deficiency diseases of their peers.

Does this mean that your children should *never* have a hamburger, cola, ice cream, or candy? No. If you have done your job well, your children will be sensible and be able to handle social situations adroitly. They will still want to go to birthday parties and proms, and hang out at the local burger joint. But this is where they will need the self-discipline, confidence, and social skills to limit the potential damage.

At home, you have an iron responsibility to ensure that the right foodstuffs are constantly available. Always have a supply of ready-to-eat fruits, vegetables, and salads. Have homemade dishes like vegetable hot-pot and ratatouille available in the fridge and freezer. Have stocks of oily fish like canned salmon, sardines, and tuna. Water should still be the main drink; try carbonated water with a twist of lemon. Unsweetened tea, iced or otherwise, is also okay. Finally, remind yourself that a child needs a role model. From the youngest age, your child will want to emulate the feeding patterns of the adults in the house.

Get your child into the habit of filling up with food at home, and preparing and taking food supplies with her when she goes out. Never have junk foods in the house. Never buy cookies, cakes, pastries, candies, hamburgers, hot dogs, ice cream, pizzas, or ready-made meals. Never have colas, fruit juices, or carbonated drinks in the house. If they are not there, the child will not make a habit of eating them.

What about condiments? It's been said that the only way to get a kid to eat his vegetables is to smother them in ketchup. If that is what works, then it is tolerable; a good quality ketchup is not such a bad condiment. The main drawback is the sugar content. Read the ingredients label and only choose the best—there are low-salt, low-sugar versions available. Better yet is to make it yourself.

Don't forget herbs and spices. They are full of healthful micronutrients (hence their pungent tastes and aromas). Get into the habit of using copious quantities of "Green" natural herbs and spices in all your dishes. Wean yourself and your family off processed sauces and table salt.

We cannot emphasize enough the importance of a healthy adolescence. Ensure that your children follow the Savanna Model, lock into place healthy habits for them, and they will be grateful to you for the rest of their long, disease-free lives.

Pregnant and Nursing Women

All we know about how our bodies work, and how our prehistoric ancestors evolved, shows that no special departure from the Savanna Model is needed during pregnancy. Sometimes women are, mistakenly, advised to load up on calcium tablets. However, our ancestors never knew anything about calcium. Certainly, we have no instincts to search out calcium-rich foods. But if that doesn't convince you, studies show that calcium supplementation does not make any difference to calcium metabolism.

The mother's body naturally meets the demand for extra calcium by three hormonal activities. First, the intestines absorb a higher percentage of calcium from everyday foods. Also, the kidneys become more efficient at recycling calcium recovered from the urine. Finally, some calcium is borrowed from the bones. Nothing that the mother eats, supplements, or does changes this process.[10] As soon as menstruation restarts, bone density steadily recovers all by itself.

Our forager ancestors had pregnancies spaced about every four years. This happened mainly through biological machinery: A woman is much less likely to conceive when breastfeeding, and she is less fertile when her body's food stores are low. The main lesson to draw from this is that it is best to space pregnancies by about four years, just like our ancient ancestors, so that the bones can recover their full health before the next pregnancy.

Your doctor will probably prescribe all kinds of dietary supplements. Know that the pregnant Bond Effect practitioner need have no fear of dietary deficiencies. (See "What About Supplements?" inset on page 109.) For example, one of the vitamins most likely to be recommended for pregnant women is folic acid because the diet of the average American woman is deficient in it. But where is folic acid found? In foliage! The Bond Effect mother naturally will absorb high levels of folic acid, as well as all the other essential nutrients for her baby, in salads and other vegetables.

On the contrary, it is even more important to not consume non-conforming foods like bad fats and bad carbohydrates. The bad fats will reappear in the fetus and in breast milk. The excess insulin levels will upset the baby's metabolism.

What about Supplements?

Many people think that it is a good idea to take supplements, particularly if they have a medical condition, but this is a very narrow way of looking at nutrition. There are thousands of compounds that are important to the harmonious functioning of the body, and they all need to be working together. It is unrealistic to think that we can compensate for dietary errors by cherry-picking this or that supplement. Worse, dosing up on one compound can have unforeseen and detrimental ramifications.

If you are eating according to the Savanna Model, what is the likelihood that you are suffering any deficiencies? The answer is, highly unlikely. You will be consuming eight times the weight of non-starchy plant food compared to the average American. So, even on plant foods with "reduced levels" of micronutrients in the soil in which they're grown, your intake will be well into the healthy intake comfort zone. The one nutrient that is hard to get this way is omega-3 essential fatty acids. In this regard, we strongly recommend eating at least one portion of oily fish per day instead of popping an omega-3 supplement.

The central tenet of the Bond Effect is that we will find all the nutrients we need by eating the right kinds of foods in the right patterns. The whole thrust of our message is to discourage people from the prevailing idea that they can avoid hard choices, keep their bad eating habits, and compensate by "taking a pill."

Finally, what about the cravings and nausea that accompany morning sickness? This is definitely a tough time for the pregnant woman. Evolutionary biologist Dr. Margie Profet opines that this sickness is nature's way of preventing women from consuming plants whose anti-nutrients might harm the fetus.[11] In addition, the fetus is already manipulating the woman's hormones to serve its own purposes, making her feel bad. What should she do? The truth is, not a lot. This is a time for going with the flow. She eats when she can and what she can bear to eat. Just relax and wait for this phase to pass. The fetus will make sure it gets all it needs, robbing the mother's own stores, if need be.

Adults in Their Thirties

This is likely to be a phase of life when health will seem good and there appears to be no need to concern yourself about the future. The reality is that it is this period of life when you need to set the scene for your later years. Bad eating habits now will lead inevitably to obesity, heart disease, and diabetes. They lay the foundation for the degenerative diseases of middle and old age—cancer, arthritis, osteoporosis, rheumatism, and even Alzheimer's.

It is at this age that the blood sugar control mechanism starts to show its age. It copes less well with the stress that we put on it. It is now that the dreaded "middle-age spread"—the bloated stomach—begins to show. This is your warning that you are pre-diabetic: Take it seriously. Change your eating pattern and relieve your body of that sugar-stress by following the guidelines in this book. But, most importantly, this is the end of the phase in which your body easily builds up bone density. Now is the time to ensure that your bone capital is at a maximum.

The Menopausal Woman

Menopausal changes start in the early forties and build up to a finality in the fifties. As with pregnancy, this is a time when a woman's hormones are undergoing a major reshuffle. It is potentially a period when Western women will have symptoms including hot flashes, irritability, hypersensitivity, depression, tension headaches, and night sweats. However, in most simple societies, these symptoms are almost unknown. Indeed, many women in the West do not suffer them, either. What makes the difference?

Not surprisingly, the main thing influencing hormonal balance is food. The bodily dysfunctions caused by dietary errors will be amplified during menopause. Controlled studies show that a diet rich in bioflavonoids and vitamin C provides relief of menopausal symptoms for many women. Where are bioflavonoids and vitamin C found? In fruits and vegetables! Just boosting the intake of fruits and vegetables is enough to dramatically reduce the disagreeable symptoms. And don't forget that bad carbohydrates and bad fats have a major effect on hormonal balances. Getting these right helps enormously, too. Eliminate dietary errors by eating according to the Savanna Model.

There are also secondary dimensions that affect women in menopause, such as the stress of the Western way of life, the psychological finality of becoming infertile, and the tension in relationships caused by changes in libido. There is a strong mind/body connection: Managing stress and moods will also help stabilize hormonal balance.

What about the long-term effects? What about osteoporosis and heart disease? These are both major problems for post-menopausal women, but only in the West. If you get your eating patterns right and get other lifestyle factors into a conforming pattern, you can get on with life and not worry about these conditions.

Finally, what about hormone replacement therapy (HRT)? HRT is sometimes prescribed to ease the symptoms of menopause. It often involves dosage of the hormone called estrogen; during menopause, the level of estrogen that the body naturally produces drops. From an ancestral health viewpoint, there is no reason why a menopausal Bond Effect practitioner should supplement with estrogen. It's a personal decision.

The Elderly

It is in the later years of life that eating in harmony with our savanna-bred natures can bring rapid relief to distressing ailments like stiff joints, arthritis, digestive upsets, and general ill health. For a great part of our lives, your body's biochemistry has sufficient "redundancy" built into its system to patch around errors of lifestyle. With old age, these margins of error disappear. Now, more than ever, it is important to harmonize how you eat with the needs of your body. When you do so, many of these troublesome maladies disappear.

Eating in accordance with the Savanna Model is the ideal and there are no other special measures to take. Just make sure that your teeth, whether original or artificial, are working efficiently. Many old people eat badly simply because they choose foods that don't need chewing. As an older person, make sure that you are eating the proper rations of fruit, salads, and vegetables. Surveys show that older people, who tend to have less efficient digestive systems, often skimp on these foods. As a result, they and their immune systems are deficient in antioxidants and other essential micronutrients. Get that right and you'll live out your years in good shape.

Vegetarians and Vegans

By "vegetarian," we mean someone who does not eat animals that have been killed, but consumes other foods of animal origin, such as dairy products and eggs. By "vegan," we mean someone who avoids foods from any animal source whatsoever. Many vegetarians and vegans make the mistake of simply eliminating animal matter from their normal, "eat anything" diet. As a result, some vegetarians and vegans are obese, have poor complexions, and suffer ill health simply because they are continuing with other bad habits. Notably, this is because they replace the animal food with increasing consumption of cereals, bread, pasta, and other complex carbohydrates. There are other errors as well, such as the use of dairy products, lentils, beans, tofu, soy protein, and bad fats and oils.

Vegetarians and vegans will find in the pages of this book exactly the right prescription for eating healthily. All you have to do is eat in accordance with the Savanna Model, ignoring the animal products where they are mentioned and choosing the vegetable alternatives instead.

Veganism can be a healthy lifestyle, provided that you carefully follow the Savanna Model consumption pattern. The secret is to eat like the gorilla, a natural vegan: Consume very high volumes of plant material, including nuts, and avoid all the bad foods that do not conform to the Savanna Model diet. Vegans need to worry about the one nutrient that is not available in their diet: Vitamin B12. The gorilla makes it in his intestine, but humans do not. (This suggests that veganism is not a natural human eating pattern.) Vegans should take supplements of vitamin B12: Just 2 micrograms per day will be enough. Vegetarians, on the other hand, will get all the B12 they need by eating eggs.

CONCLUSION

Adopting the Savanna Model diet can seem like a daunting task initially. However, as you gradually get used to replacing grains, legumes, sugars, and other non-conforming foods with leafy greens, vegetables, fruits, and nuts, you will find that it is not so difficult after all. As an added benefit, you will feel healthier and more energetic, and you will not be plagued by the Western diseases that affect so many others. Adopt the diet at your own pace; perhaps start by replacing just one meal a day, or follow the three-stage plan I have outlined in this chapter. Consider what are the best foods to eat if you are pregnant, have children, are menopausal, or are vegetarian/vegan. If you have a lapse, that is okay. Continue to look to the future and enjoy the rest of your days healthy and disease-free.

Conclusion

Healthy Lifespan
and the Best of Both Worlds

I n this guide, you have been given an overview into the lives of our relatives: The foragers and hunter-gatherers of the savanna. They followed specific patterns of eating, sleeping, and activity that we would do well to abide by today. Habits such as rising with the sun, employing themselves, and frequent walking allowed the foragers to live satisfying lives free from lifestyle disease. The type of food they ate was most important to their lifestyle. They sought plant food that was high in alkalizing elements, micronutrients, fiber, and potassium, and that was low-sodium, low-glycemic, and low-insulinemic. Plant foods were supplemented with meat and the rare dose of honey, but the foragers ate no grains, dairy, or processed foods—foods that dominate our marketplace today.

It may seem silly to recommend following the diets and lifestyles of our ancestors that lived millions of years ago. Sometimes people say to me, "Ah, but we live so much longer than they did, don't we!"...as though there were no old people in a forager band. This is rubbish. In fact, as we have seen, the grandparent generation was vital to the survival of the human species.

OLD AGE AND CLIFF-EDGE MORTALITY

That is not to say the foragers could elude death. However, the elderly certainly were not unhealthy. Every few days or weeks, a forager band had to walk 10 to 15 miles to the next campsite. Everyone had to make that walk, including the grandparents! That is the normal human condition: To stay fully functioning until the end of our days.

But a point will come in an old forager person's life where he announces: "I don't think I can make that long walk to the next campsite..." He will lie down, the band will make him comfortable, and, over a few days, the old person fades away. This is known as "cliff-edge mortality."

These people do not die of any identifiable disease, like cancer or heart disease. No, on the contrary, *they die of old age!* That is to say, all parts of the body have aged to the point where everything shuts down at the same time.

Even today, some people of extreme age die like this. It's just that now, doctors have to certify a *cause* of death—and "old age" is no longer seen as a valid cause. Be that as it may, the vast majority of centenarians and "super-centenarians" (those over the age of 110) live a forager-like end-of-life where there is compression of morbidity. This means that any lifestyle diseases, like heart disease or respiratory disease, are not present until the very last few months of life. In other words, just like foragers, they have very long, healthy lifespans.

In contrast, the average American, the one who has lived the modern dysfunctional lifestyle, can expect to spend the last *eight years* of life "disabled" by disease.[1] Obesity rates amongst the old have rocketed from 11 percent in 1991 to over 30 percent in 2009,[2,3] and almost all of the elderly will be on a variety of powerful medications.

OTHER CAUSES OF DEATH IN FORAGERS

Forager mothers were fatalistic: 40 to 50 percent of their babies died before they were three years old. Many of these deaths happened because something went wrong with the birth or, occasionally, the baby might have had some disability. After that, infectious diseases like dysentery and malaria, as well as accidents and predators, carried them off. Of course, this high rate of mortality in the early years dragged down the figures for life expectancy, figures which are still misunderstood by the general public (and by many health practitioners, who should know better).

Once this dangerous time was survived, the next most deadly time was for young men. Some 20 to 25 percent died in battle. Warfare, feuds, and vendettas with neighboring forager bands were an ever-present feature of our ancient ancestors' lives.

At any point in their lives, foragers could have succumbed to accidents and predation. They would fall out of baobab trees while on a honey expedition, stab themselves with a poison arrow, suffer a snake bite, or be attacked by a leopard.

After all is said and done, some 25 percent of the population would survive all these vicissitudes to die of the old age I spoke of earlier.

MODERN CAUSES OF DEATH

Americans die, first and foremost, of lifestyle diseases which are, in descending order of importance: Cardiovascular disease (28 percent), cancer (23 percent), iatrogenic (caused by medical treatment) causes (10 percent), respiratory disease (6 percent), and then a long tail of various other sicknesses and illnesses.[4]

Iatrogenic causes—Greek for "the doctor did it"—are a prevalent cause of death. Some 250,000 people die each year because of their medical treatment.[5] It is the third-leading cause of death for Americans. The problem is not bad doctors; it is that, given the incredible complexity of modern medicine, things will go wrong.

Diabetes doesn't appear in the list because sufferers mostly die of a complication caused by diabetes—usually cardiovascular disease, but also kidney disease or even cancer.

THE BEST OF BOTH WORLDS

The information provided in this guide holds out an inspiring prize—we can have the best of both worlds. We can avoid the lifestyle diseases of modern industrial societies, and we can avoid the infectious diseases, mishaps, and murder that foragers are subject to.

It is often said that the fate of man is to grow old, to get sick, and to die. But this is not entirely true—the "sick" stage is not inevitable! The moral is this: Whether we age well, or age badly, is largely up to us and whether we adopt the way of living and eating that nature has intended for us all along.

Population Studies Supporting The Paleo Lifestyle

A s we saw, humans fanned out from Africa some 2,000 generations ago until, by 15,000 years ago, they had installed themselves in all habitable parts of the planet. As a result, this tropical creature, *Homo sapiens,* now lives in places that are *not* tropical. Moreover, these groups were obliged to change their lifestyles in order to fit in with local circumstances.

Today, the planet is like a huge laboratory with experiments going on in different parts. It is an ideal opportunity to statistically study how different lifestyles affect health and longevity. Let's look at some examples of interesting populations to see how their lifestyle and diet has changed from the Savanna Model and what effect this mismatch has had on their health.

LIFE EXPECTANCY AND "HEALTH EXPECTANCY"

A good starting point for analysis is to examine countrywide statistics for death rates and the *reasons* for death. National governments collect these figures and international bodies like the World Health Organization (WHO) collate them. Life expectancy is the factor that is most often paraded as an indication of how well a country is doing.

The figures most bandied about are for "life expectancy at birth." This means the average number of years every baby born alive might be expected to live. In Pleistocene times, or even with the San today, 30 percent of babies would die within the first year. This drags down the averages for "life expectancy *at birth,*"particularly in the underdeveloped world. For this reason, researchers often look at life expectancy at a later age, often at age fifteen. This gives the average number of years a fifteen-year-old is expected to live. This produces some surprising and useful results: We find that once an individual from a poor country has made it safely to fifteen years old, he can expect to live as long, or even longer, than his counterparts in industrialized societies.

For example, fifteen-year-old boys can expect to live to the age of 81.4 in Hong Kong, 80.5 in Japan, 78.3 in Greece, but only 77.1 in the United States.[1] Women live longer than men in all countries and the proportions are similar: Fifteen-year-old girls can expect to live to the age of 87.0 in Hong Kong, 86.9 in Japan, 83.3 in

Greece, but only 81.8 in the U.S. The Japanese overall have the longest life expectancy in the world, closely followed by people living in Hong Kong.

Even if we measure life expectancy at *birth,* Chinese boys born in the Shanghai province have a life expectancy of 75.7 years, while American boys at birth have a life expectancy of 71.8.[2] Shanghai baby girls can expect to live for 79.2 years, but American baby girls can only expect 78.6 years of life.

The information gets even more interesting as we drill down to find out what diseases are prevalent in certain countries and what diseases their populations die of. Deliberately, we go back in time to sample the conditions when people's lifestyles were much more traditional. For example, in 1960, for every 100,000 men, 466 Americans died of heart disease, whereas only forty-eight Greeks died of it. Greeks were five times more likely to die of a stroke than an Egyptian. Britons were 1.5 times as likely to die of cancer as a Yugoslav.[3] In 1978, Norwegian women were five times more likely to suffer a hip fracture than a Spanish woman.[4] In 1954, Japanese women had a very low incidence of breast cancer— just four deaths per 10,000—compared to 18.5 deaths in the U.S.; an American man was twenty times more likely to die of prostate cancer than a Japanese man.[5]

There is little correlation between health and wealth. Japan and the U.S. are both rich countries, but poor countries can be healthy, too. In 1978, Albania was the poorest country in Europe with an annual income of only $380 per person. In spite of that, an Albanian man was half as likely to die of coronary heart disease as a British man,[6] who earned some thirty-three times as much at $12,775 per year on average![7]

There is another often-used measure of well-being known as "health expectancy"—this is the number of years that a person can expect to live "in full health." Based on this measure, the Japanese have the highest health expectancy of 74.5 years.[8] In comparison, the British come in fourteenth with 71.7 years and Americans come in twenty-fourth with only 70.0 years. In other words, you are likely to die earlier and spend more time disabled (on average) if you are an American.

Statistics like this give us plenty to ponder. What is so special about the Greeks, the Japanese, and the Hong Kong Chinese that they live longer (and in better shape) than Americans? Why are some people more vulnerable to cancers, heart disease, strokes, and osteoporosis than others? There is now a massive body of research to identify how different populations' lifestyles influence their life and health expectancy. We will look at the knowledge obtained for a few populations to see how the evidence builds up. To get the best contrast, we have chosen some extreme cases.

ESKIMOS

As our species spread out around the world, it settled in even the most inhospitable regions. The Eskimos were originally Siberians who got pushed across the Bering Strait by population pressures. They arrived in Alaska 6,000 years ago and found the land already occupied by the American Indians, who had migrated there several thousand years earlier. The only available territory was the land that the American Indians had shied away from—the unimaginably difficult Arctic regions of Alaska and Canada.

The Eskimos live in the most extreme of unfavorable environments. It is either cool, cold, or extremely cold most of the time. However, they have no biological special adaptation for these temperatures—the Eskimos are still tropical creatures. They can only live inside the Arctic Circle by insulating themselves from it. This was possible once some Siberian ancestor had worked out how to kill and skin a large furry animal and tailor it into a weather-tight garment. Like astronauts who are obliged to wear spacesuits to work in the vacuum of outer space, so the Eskimos have to cocoon themselves in animal furs to live in the Arctic cold.

The Eskimos' main activity is hunting and traveling, but they also spend quite a lot of time eating, sleeping, and loafing about.[9] In the depths of winter, just warming up the air they breathe takes 1,000 calories. They eat much of their meat frozen, and that costs their bodies another 300 calories just to thaw it out. Oxford University professor/explorer Hugh MacDonald Sinclair specialized in studying the Eskimo diet at a time when there were still many Eskimos living the traditional way. In 1953, he estimated that, in winter, the average Eskimo needs to consume about 4,500 calories per day.[10]

In Eskimo society, contrary to the Savanna Model, hunting is not a luxury but a necessity. It is virtually the only source of food—at no time is gathering an option as a mainstay. Men are still the driving force in the hunt, although often the women come along and help. Even so, in complete contrast to the Savanna Model, the women and children are highly dependent on their men to feed them. The women are occupied with the domestic chores of skinning the kill, preparing the food, and making clothes and other artifacts.

The Eskimo Diet

How did the Eskimos feed themselves? Today, the Eskimo has the double-edged "benefit" of modern civilization, so we have to go back to quite old studies, archives, and records. Dr. Anne Keenleyside is a Canadian researcher with special interest in paleopathology, the analysis of ancient bones. She found that, with virtually no vegetation in their environment and winter temperatures dropping to below −40°F, the Eskimos had to rely almost entirely on animal sources for their food.[11] Dr. Keenleyside and many other researchers have built up a picture of the traditional Eskimo feeding pattern. Eskimos hunted fish, seal, whale, walrus, musk ox, caribou, polar bears, wolves, birds, rabbits, ducks, and geese. They ate every part of the animal—brains, blood, intestines, and even the feces. On occasion, the women would gather eggs, crabs, mollusks, and shellfish.

The Eskimos were particularly fond of the rather sour contents of the caribou paunch.[12] These are the partly digested remains of lichens and mosses. They cut the blubber off the kill for use as lighting oil and other external uses. They ate most animal food raw, sometimes after considerable putrefaction. Other foods, particularly seal meat, were eaten frozen. Some foods were lightly cooked over a seal-oil lamp or boiled or roasted. Because the Eskimo lives above the tree line, a campfire was a rare luxury fed by dried seaweed and other dried plant remains.[13] In times of plenty, the Eskimo could consume prodigious amounts of meat: 9 lbs in a day has been measured as a normal occurrence. At such times they drank prodigious amounts of water, too—which is a direct result of eating an excess of protein (see "Alkalizing" section in Chapter 1 and "Acid-alkali Balance" section in the Owner's Manual). The kidneys needed to flush out the overabundant amino acids (proteins).

It was only in the short summer that the Eskimo ate any plant food. The treeless plains of the Arctic have a permanently frozen subsoil, known as tundra, and no plants grow more than knee-high. The women would forage for berries, roots, stalks, buds, and leaves. They gathered some kinds of algae and seaweed, too. It is estimated, however, that plant food represented no more than about 5 percent of the diet, even during the growing season.

The muscle meat of seal and whale shares similar characteristics with our ancestral wild game—there is little "marbling," or fat permeating the muscle. The small amount of muscle fat and the visible fat (blubber) are particularly rich in essential fatty acids (EFAs), notably the omega-3 fish oil called eicosapentaenoic acid (EPA). As we saw in "The Power of Essential Fatty Acids" in Chapter 3, our modern industrial diets are starved of such omega-3 fish oils, whereas the Eskimo has a superabundance of them.

Dr. George Mann, in a report for the U.S. National Defense Committee in 1962, stated that by eating all the animal parts, the Eskimo obtained enough of the "classic" micronutrients to survive, including vitamin C.[14] This might come as a surprise, since we think of vitamin C as only coming from plants. However, the skin and guts of animals like seal and caribou are also rich in this vitamin. On the other hand, the Eskimo diet was very deficient in "background" micronutrients.

Calcium consumption was huge—over 2,000 mg per day.[15] Protein intake was very high and the fat and oil intake was high.[16] However, the types of fat are of key importance: The Eskimo diet was very low in saturated fat, high (as we saw) in omega-3 fish oils, and quite high in cholesterol; there were virtually no unhealthy trans fatty acids. The Eskimos' intake of fiber, carbohydrates, and sugars was almost nonexistent, although they got some glycogen (a kind of animal carbohydrate) from the meat. Canadian researcher Kang-Jey Ho estimates that 50 percent of energy came from fat, 35 percent from protein, and 15 percent from glycogen.[17] Most notably, there was virtually no plant food, no soluble fiber, nor the myriad of micronutrients that only plant foods can provide. Below, we will look at the health effects of such a diet.

Eskimo Health

The Eskimos first attracted attention because of an anomaly: In spite of their high-fat, high-meat diet, they had no cardiovascular disease, thromboses, or strokes; they had low blood pressure and good cholesterol levels.[18] In fact, it was too much of a good thing. Their blood was slow to clot when needed (known as a prolonged "bleeding time") and they suffered from enduring nose-bleeds. These discoveries led researchers to find the vital role of the various fatty acids in manipulating body biochemistry. The Eskimos did not suffer from cancer, diabetes, multiple sclerosis, or arthritis. Neither did they suffer from vitamin C deficiency (scurvy) or from vitamin D deficiency (rickets); nor did they get appendicitis or dental caries (cavities).

On the other hand, the Eskimos aged fast: They became wizened and shriveled so that a fifty-year-old looked more like an eighty-year-old. It is speculated that this is due to the lack of antioxidants in the diet—and that this is an example of the "free radical" theory of aging.[19]

We can learn something from their high calcium intake of up to 2,000 mg per day. In spite of this megadose of calcium, the Eskimos suffered from bone demineralization and osteoporosis.[20] Doesn't this go against all we are told today? This should make us question a major nutritional doctrine—that we have only to swallow calcium by the bucketful to avoid osteoporosis. In fact, good bone health is a very complex matter, easily upset by a myriad of lifestyle factors, of which calcium intake is almost irrelevant. (See "Bone Health" section in Chapter 3.)

Today, the Eskimos suffer the same fate as other hunter-gatherers who adopt the Western lifestyle: High rates of obesity, heart disease, diabetes, rotten teeth, and high mortality. Life expectancy has dropped even lower.

THE JAPANESE

We are all familiar with rice, the so-called staple of the Japanese diet. We say "so-called" because there are two misconceptions about rice. First, the Japanese did not eat that much of it—even as recently as 1998, daily consumption of rice was just 6 oz. And although rice retains a hallowed place in Japanese hearts, it is regarded as a poor man's food to be replaced by plant foods whenever possible.[21]

Traditionally, the Japanese are Buddhists and, as such, they did not eat animals at all. However, they did eat fish, often raw. By Western standards, it was a high consumption, around 90 g (3.15 oz) per person per day (four times as much as the average American). From this, they got a high consumption of omega-3 fish oil, notably the essential fatty acid eicosapentaenoic acid (EPA). Even so, their overall consumption of fat was very low—no more than 10 percent of total calories—which is much lower than the U.S. Department of Agriculture recommended (but rarely achieved) maximum of 30 percent.

The largest percentage of their fat came from rapeseed (canola) oil. East Asians have cultivated rapeseed for millennia, and the Japanese have used rapeseed oil in frugal amounts for at least 2,000 years. To a lesser extent, they used soybean oil. Consumption of saturated fats, hydrogenated fats, and trans fatty acids was almost zero.

The idea of dairy farming had never reached Japan and dairy products never formed part of their traditional diet. Rice was the staple and other cereals were virtually unknown. The Japanese traditionally did not eat wheat, barley, rye, or oats. They did not eat potatoes, either. So, when we say that Japanese consumption of rice was 6 oz per day, that is it: No other low-grade starch fillers such as bread, pasta, pizza, or French fries existed in their diet.

But all that has changed now. The first McDonald's arrived in 1972 and through the 1970s and 1980s, the Japanese diet rapidly became Westernized. The younger generations are now experiencing the same harmful impacts on health as their American counterparts. In older populations, the dietary transition has contributed to the rapid increase in Alzheimer's disease rates in Japan.[22]

The Japanese traditionally had to husband their resources and they ate much more sparingly than is our custom in the West. They had a high consumption of salt (mostly from soy sauce) of 12.4 g per person per day in 2010. This is a great deal worse than government recommendations of 6.2 g per day maximum.[23] The Japanese also smoke a lot: Up until the late 1970s, 70 percent of men and 45 percent of women smoked some form of tobacco.[24] Since then, these rates have declined steadily to 30 percent of men and 10 percent of women in 2015. [24]

Japanese Longevity and Health

Japanese men have a life expectancy four years greater than Americans and their health expectancy is 4.5 years longer than Americans. But studies show that this only applies as long as the Japanese stay in Japan and eat the traditional Japanese diet. When Japanese migrate to America and/or adopt the American way of life, including its diet, their life expectancy drops to the American norm and they get the same diseases.[25] This suggests that Japanese health and longevity are not about genes but about the way the Japanese live their lives, notably the foods they eat and do not eat.

At home, by a fluke of culture, geography, and luck, the Japanese have hit on a good lifestyle, but even so, it is not perfect. For example, they smoke too much and they consume too much salt. More than in most other countries, the Japanese die of strokes and heart disease. The diet of raw fish means that they absorb the live eggs and larvae of intestinal parasites, so that worm infestations of the gut, virtually unknown in the West, are quite common in Japan.

Within the general statistics for Japan are buried even more startling results.

The archipelago (group of islands) of Okinawa is remote from the Japanese mainland and its population has an even more enviable record for health and longevity. They have one of the highest proportions of centenarians in the world: Their chances of living to 100 are twelve times those of an American. Not only do the people live a long time, but the elderly live in good health as well. In a study of thirty-nine 80-year-olds, 90 percent were fully functional human beings without any disability; only three had impaired hearing and only four had fading eyesight.[26]

A study carried out in the remote and tiny Okinawan island of Kohama found that the inhabitants eat even more fish, 144 g (about 5 oz), and far less salt, about 6 g per day, than their mainland neighbors.[27] They eat seaweed and herbaceous plants and also sweet potato and tofu (soybean curd). They have adopted some Chinese practices from nearby Taiwan, eating some pork and drinking green tea. And they exercise a lot: 95 percent of the eighty-year-olds studied led active lives, working long hours every day in their fish-farming paddies.

The Okinawans are a poor people, but even the poorest precinct has better longevity—two years more—than the already stellar performance of Japan as a whole.[28] They have the lowest incidence of cardiovascular disease in all of Japan, even though they smoke the same amount. At age fifty-nine, only 8 percent of the population had high blood pressure, 2.3 percent had heart disease, and 1.2 percent had diabetes. These figures are two to three times better than mainland Japan. However, the Okinawans had *double* the incidence of senile dementia. Their high tofu consumption could be an explanantion.[29]

The remarkable health and longevity of the Okinawans has generated a number of diet programs. However, as a comparison with the Owner's Manual, there is still room for improvement.

THE CRETANS

Similar observations have been made with the peoples of the Mediterranean northern rim. The people of the Greek island of Crete had one of the highest life expectancies in the world, in spite of a hard lifestyle. Indeed, although half a world away, there are many similarities with the Okinawan way of life. The Cretans ate frugally; they ate fish but virtually no meat (just the occasional goat's meat, as beef was nonexistent); they ate plenty of plant food, notably a salad-green called purslane; and they consumed very little dairy, pastries, or sugars. Unlike the Okinawans, they ate bread—a rough-ground, whole-wheat variety—and they had a moderate fat consumption through the sparing use of olive oil in the kitchen. They also had an extraordinary custom: For the Cretan, traditional breakfast often consisted of a small amount of olive oil downed in one gulp, and that was it until lunch time. Wine was also commonly drunk, but in moderation.

These people were poor and complained that they felt hungry most of the time. They were obliged to be physically active on their land until an advanced age. Yet, the Cretans had the longest lifespan in Europe and their incidences of heart disease, colon cancer, high blood pressure, osteoporosis, and diabetes were much lower than the peoples of northern Europe and North America.

American researcher Ancel Keys, who first investigated the fabled Cretan longevity and health in the 1950s, wrote a book about his findings, which later became popular as the so-called Mediterranean diet.[30] But this Mediterranean diet has nothing in common with the kind of meal you will find in an Italian, Spanish, or French restaurant. It contains no spaghetti, paella, pizza, or French fries; even less does it contain their rich cheeses and cream sauces.

With the advance of prosperity and the crumbling of old traditions, the Cretans have begun to adopt Western eating habits, and their deterioration in health is being documented.

Testing the Cretan Diet

In the meantime, the baton has passed to researchers who investigated the Mediterranean diet with well-controlled clinical trials. These trials are studies where large groups of people are divided into two test groups. One group is the "experimental" group: They are given the new diet to eat over several years. The second group is the "control" group: They continue to eat their normal diet. At the beginning of the study, both groups are tested for various health indicators, such as blood pressure, cholesterol levels, weight, and so on. They are then retested at intervals as time goes by. Often these studies go on for five or ten years, during which there will also be some deaths.

Thousands of clinical trials have tested various hypotheses about food and how it affects health and lifespan. The results of such studies give us very clear indications as to what is right for human beings to eat and what is not. We have not the space here to go into the detail of all these studies. We will therefore cite one powerful example and then give a summary of the overall picture that the collection of studies paints for us.

Under chief researcher Professor Serge Renaud, the Lyon Diet Heart Study published in 1994 involved a group of 606 heart attack patients living in Lyon, France. The group was equally divided into a "control group" and an "experimental group."[31] The control group followed the conventional advice of the hospital dietitians based on the American Heart Association (AHA) diet. The experimental group was told to adopt a Cretan-type diet: More green vegetables and root vegetables, more fish, less meat, and replace beef, pork, and lamb with poultry, no day without fruit, and replace butter and cream with a special margarine made from canola (rapeseed) oil. Olive oil and/or canola oil replaced all other fats. Moderate wine consumption was allowed.

After twenty-seven months, the experiment was stopped early: Members of the control group on the AHA diet were dying at a much faster rate than those on the Cretan diet. There were sixteen deaths on the AHA diet, compared to just three on the Cretan diet. The AHA group was also suffering a much higher rate of second heart attacks: There were seventeen non-fatal heart attacks, compared to just five on the Cretan diet.

It is not as though the AHA diet was bad—it was certainly better than how the patients were eating before the start of the study—but the Cretan diet proved to be exceptionally superior even to the conventional dietary treatment recommended by the American Heart Association. The committee charged with looking after the welfare of the groups swiftly decided to stop the trial early so that the AHA group of patients could benefit from the study's insights and adopt the Cretan diet if they so desired.

SUMMARY—POPULATION STUDY CLUES

Researchers have carried out thousands of similar clinical studies on a huge range of different dietary factors. It is an exciting story in itself, but it is not the purpose of this book to relate them in detail. However, the results of such studies do fill in some important gaps in the "Owner's Manual." We have distilled these results into the following generalized summaries. They highlight the foods linked to disease and the foods linked to health. This is a broad-brush approach, but the circumstantial evidence is pointing strongly to lifestyle patterns close to our ancestral, naturally adapted ones.

CLINICAL STUDIES SUMMARY OF HELPFUL FOODS		
FOODS	**DISEASES PROMOTED**	**DISEASES THWARTED**
Fruit		Arthritis
Non-starchy vegetables		Bowel diseases
Salads		Cancers
Tubers (non-starchy)		Constipation
Berries	None	Diabetes
Nuts (moderation)		Heart disease
Seafood and oily fish (moderation)		High blood pressure
Wild animal protein (moderation)		Indigestion
Low-fat poultry (moderation)		Infectious diseases
		Obesity
		Osteoporosis

CLINICAL STUDIES SUMMARY OF UNHELPFUL FOODS		
FOODS	**DISEASES PROMOTED**	**DISEASES THWARTED**
Bulk vegetable oils	Allergies	
Dairy products	Autoimmune diseases	
Farmed "red" meat	Cancers	
Grains	Constipation	
Saturated fats	Heart disease	None
Hydrogenated fats	High blood pressure	
Trans fats	Indigestion	
Sugars	Infectious diseases	
Starchy vegetables	Obesity	
Meat (high-meat diet)	Osteoporosis	
	Stroke	

Appendix B

Paleo-Conforming Recipes

Most of us try to do the right thing by our children and spouses, especially when it comes to feeding them. But we are confused by the conflicting messages. We are overwhelmed by the plethora of diet books and cookery manuals claiming to show us the way to health and happiness.

In this guidebook, we have brought clarity to the confusion. The solution is none other than feeding ourselves the way Mother Nature intended! That way, we avoid stressing our bodies with foods it was never designed to handle. You will draw comfort from the knowledge that, by preparing food the way we explain in this guide, you are building the foundations for long, healthy lives.

The Paleo way of life does not need you to eat in an outlandish way. Your dinner guests will be surprised to find that they have been eating what seem like conventional dishes. Only you will know what subtle, yet vital changes in ingredients—and in cooking—you have made.

When eating the Paleo way, we mostly keep it simple. There is very little in the way of processed foods; we just use generic ingredients in their natural state. Nevertheless, it takes a while to retrain one's habits and also to discover how to prepare food that is in conformity with the Paleo principles. For example, people usually find it hard to give up bread, breakfast cereals, and desserts. But you do not need to! It is possible to create conforming alternatives.

To give you an idea, we have extracted some recipes from Nicole Bond's *Paleo Harvest* cookbook. We have included bread and cereal alternatives, salads, vegetable-based dishes, meat and fish-based dishes, soups and stews, and even desserts. These are mostly straightforward recipes, using easy-to-find ingredients. Enjoy!

BREAD, CEREAL & PASTRY ALTERNATIVES

ALMOND FLOUR BREAD

This is a basic bread. It is easy to make and has a very satisfactory taste and toasting quality. The xanthan gum provides the "stickiness" that gluten would otherwise provide.

YIELD: 15–20 SLICES

5 large omega-3 eggs

$2^{1}/_{4}$ cups almond flour

2 tablespoons olive oil

2 tablespoons red wine vinegar

$^{1}/_{2}$ teaspoon salt, or to taste

$^{3}/_{4}$ teaspoon baking soda

1 teaspoon xanthan gum

Olive oil spray

1. Preheat the oven to 340°F (170°C).

2. Combine all dough ingredients in a food processor and, using the blade, mix them to obtain a smooth consistency.

3. Spray a loaf pan (about 8 x 4 x 3 inches) with the olive oil and fill with the mixture.

4. Bake for about 35 minutes. Check the center for doneness by inserting a toothpick in the center. The bread is done if the toothpick comes out clean.

5. Allow the bread to cool down before serving.

QUICHE AND PIZZA DOUGH

This wheat-free dough can be used as the basis for many dishes, including pizza or Broccoli Quiche (see page 136). It is a versatile and tasty basic dough.

YIELD: 10-INCH QUICHE OR PIZZA

2 omega-3 eggs

3 tablespoons olive oil

1 tablespoon red wine vinegar

$1/4$ teaspoon baking powder

$1/4$ teaspoon salt

1 cup almond flour

2 tablespoons coconut flour

3 tablespoons flax seed flour

2 tablespoons chia or sesame seeds

1. Beat the eggs in a medium-size mixing bowl with an electric hand mixer until thoroughly mixed.

2. Blend in all other ingredients, until you obtain a pastry of thick consistency. Knead with your hands on a sheet of wax paper and form into a ball.

3. Chill dough for an hour before using as directed in your recipe of choice.

PALEO MUESLI

Traditional muesli, which has oat flakes as a base, is off-limits.
Here, we replace the oats with a nourishing blend of conforming
alternatives, notably chia seeds. You can adjust the ingredients
to your preference by adding other nuts, like pine nuts or
finely chopped walnuts and pecan nuts.

YIELD: 6 SERVINGS

Muesli:

$1/_2$ cup chia seeds

2 tablespoons raisins

2 tablespoons sesame seeds

2 tablespoons pumpkin seeds

2 tablespoons chopped almonds

3 tablespoons shredded coconut, unsweetened

5 tablespoons xylitol, or more or less to taste

1 teaspoon ground cinnamon

Add per portion:

7 tablespoons almond milk, hazelnut milk,
or coconut milk

Optional (per portion):

1 teaspoon vanilla extract

1 tablespoon dried goji berries

2 tablespoons fresh chopped fruit

1. Combine the muesli ingredients and store in a jar.

2. In order to prepare one serving, place $1/_4$ cup of the combined muesli ingredients in an individual bowl.

3. Stir in 7 tablespoons of nut milk to one serving and wait about 10 minutes for the muesli to thicken.

4. Stir the mixture thoroughly and enhance, if desired, with vanilla extract, goji berries, or fresh chopped fruit before serving.

STARTERS & SALADS

"POTATO" SALAD

This is a yummy dish with an uncanny resemblance in taste and texture to a great potato salad. But this recipe (with no potato) is fully Paleo-conforming. Eat as much as you like. You may wish to adjust the quantities of the mustard, mayonnaise, and oil to taste.

YIELD: 2–3 SERVINGS AS A MAIN DISH,
4–6 SERVINGS AS A STARTER

1 cauliflower head (about 1$^1/_2$ pounds),
divided into small florets

1 tablespoon Dijon mustard

3 tablespoons mayonnaise*

2 tablespoons canola oil

1 medium onion, finely chopped

3 celery stalks, finely chopped

4 sprigs fresh parsley, finely chopped

2 omega-3 eggs, hard-boiled and finely chopped

Freshly ground black pepper, to taste

1. Steam cauliflower florets for about 10 minutes, or until tender but still crunchy. Set aside to cool.

2. In a large salad bowl, combine the mustard, mayonnaise, and oil.

3. Stir in the chopped onion, celery, and parsley.

4. Add the cauliflower florets and coat well with the onion mixture.

5. Carefully fold the chopped eggs into the cauliflower salad. Season with pepper to taste.

6. Serve immediately or chill before serving.

*Ensure your mayonnaise is Paleo-conforming: The original—and best—mayonnaise is made only from olive or canola oil, eggs, and maybe some lemon juice and mustard. If buying ready-made mayonnaise from a store, try to find a product that conforms as closely as possible to these ingredients.

ARTIST'S SALAD

This exotic salad has been served across several five-star hotels in Mediterranean resorts. It is a simple and refreshing dish that can be eaten on its own or as an accompaniment to a larger meal.

YIELD: 4 SERVINGS

5 tablespoons olive oil

3 tablespoons lemon juice

2 cups roughly chopped fresh arugula leaves

2 cups roughly chopped fresh cilantro leaves

3 cups thinly-sliced mushrooms

2 cherry tomatoes, cut in half

1. In a small mixing bowl, combine olive oil and lemon juice. Set aside.

2. Put the arugula, cilantro, and mushrooms in a medium-size salad bowl. Add the olive oil-lemon vinaigrette to taste and toss well.

3. Serve immediately on four individual plates and decorate each serving with one half of a cherry tomato.

VEGETABLE DISHES

BOHEMIAN RED CABBAGE (ROTKRAUT)

This is a delicious dish that has its origins in Central Europe. Traditionally, this dish is cooked for up to 90 minutes, until the cabbage is really limp. However, nutritionally speaking, the less time the cabbage is cooked, the better. Try cooking for no more than 30 minutes. Bohemian Red Cabbage is particularly well accompanied by a portion of game, such as venison or pheasant.

YIELD: 4 SERVINGS

1 red cabbage (about 2 pounds), thinly shredded

1 tablespoon olive oil

1 medium red onion, thinly chopped

2 tablespoons caraway seeds

$1/2$ cup balsamic vinegar

$1^1/_2$ tablespoons xylitol, or to taste

1 teaspoon allspice

1 green apple, unpeeled and grated

Salt, to taste

Freshly ground black pepper, to taste

1. Steam the cabbage for about 10 minutes. Drain and set aside.

2. Heat the olive oil in a large saucepan over medium heat and sauté the onion until soft and translucent, but not brown.

3. Add the caraway seeds and sauté briefly. Stir in the vinegar, xylitol, and allspice and sauté for another 2 minutes.

4. Mix in the grated apple and sauté another 2 minutes.

5. Add the steamed cabbage. Season with salt and pepper to taste. Stir thoroughly, to coat the cabbage evenly with all the ingredients.

6. Cover and bring slowly to a boil. Simmer on very low heat for 20 to 30 minutes, stirring once in a while to avoid the cabbage sticking to the pan.

7. Adjust the seasoning, if necessary, and check for doneness. The cabbage should be very tender and soft. Serve hot.

TOMATO SAUCE PROVENÇALE

This highly flavored tomato sauce makes a fine condiment that complements many dishes, such as Broccoli Quiche (see page 136). It can be served hot or cold.

YIELD: ABOUT 1¹/₄ CUPS

1 pound ripe tomatoes

Olive oil spray

1 medium onion, finely chopped

3 medium cloves garlic, crushed

1 teaspoon dried Herbes de Provence,
or Italian seasoning

2 bay leaves

Salt, to taste

Freshly ground black pepper, to taste

2 tablespoons chopped fresh parsley

1. In a medium-size bowl, pour boiling water over the tomatoes. Set aside for 1 minute. Drain the tomatoes, peel off the skin, cut in quarters, seed, and chop. Set aside.

2. Spray a medium-size, non-stick frying pan with the olive oil and sauté the onion over medium heat until soft and translucent, but not brown. Add the garlic and sauté for 2 minutes.

3. Add the chopped tomatoes, the Herbes de Provence, the bay leaves, and salt and pepper to taste.

4. Cook uncovered over medium heat. When most of the liquid has evaporated, reduce the heat. Simmer, uncovered, stirring frequently, until the tomatoes start to stick to the pan. This may take 50 to 60 minutes.

5. Mix in the parsley. Serve hot, chilled, or set aside for your favorite recipe.

ORIENTAL ZUCCHINI QUICK FIX

A curry is often a good way to spice up bland veggies (like zucchini). Here, by the judicious use of other Eastern spices and condiments, we conjure up a dish redolent of the Orient. Since this is meant to be a quick fix, we focus on the use of several ready-prepared ingredients, but nothing stops you from substituting fresh. This dish is best used as a side dish and tastes its best the day after its preparation.

YIELD: 4 SERVINGS

Olive oil spray

1 cup frozen chopped onion

2 teaspoons ready-made chopped garlic

1 teaspoon ready-made chopped ginger

2–3 teaspoons red curry paste (Thai or similar mild), to taste

$1/_2$ cup coconut milk

2 teaspoons light soy sauce

2 pounds zucchini, cut into bite-size pieces

2 teaspoons lemon juice

Ground black pepper, to taste

1. Spray a large frying pan (or wok) with the oil and sauté the onion over medium heat, until soft and translucent, but not brown.

2. Mix in the garlic and ginger. Sauté all together for 2 minutes.

3. Blend in the curry paste, coconut milk, and soy sauce.

4. Add the zucchini to the pan and coat with the sauce.

5. Cover and bring slowly to a boil. Simmer for about 30 minutes, or until the zucchini are tender.

6. Season with the lemon juice and pepper to taste, and serve hot.

BROCCOLI QUICHE

In the early days, we thought that we would have to give up pastry-based dishes. Now, with the discovery of how to make them safely, we are delighted that we can now consume a proper, conforming quiche. This dish will be popular with everybody; it is one of our favorites.

YIELD: 10-INCH QUICHE

1 recipe quiche and pizza dough (see page 129)

³/₄ pound fresh broccoli, cut into bite-size florets

3 omega-3 eggs

6–8 tablespoons homemade Tomato Sauce Provençale
(see page 134)

2 pinches nutmeg

5–10 drops Tabasco sauce, or to taste

Salt, to taste

Ground black pepper, to taste

2 tablespoons chopped fresh parsley

Olive oil spray

1. Preheat oven to 340°F (170°C).

2. Steam broccoli florets for about 5 minutes. The broccoli should stay crunchy. Set aside.

3. Beat the eggs with an electric hand mixer in a medium-size mixing bowl. Stir in the tomato sauce, enough to obtain the desired thickness. Season with nutmeg, Tabasco sauce, and salt and pepper to taste.

4. Combine the egg mixture with the broccoli. Add the parsley and set aside.

5. Spray a round 10-inch baking dish with the olive oil.

6. By patting with a small spatula, spread out the quiche and pizza dough in the baking dish, leaving a rim around the edge about 1 inch high. Prick the bottom of the dough with a fork. Bake in the oven for about 8 minutes, until the dough is set.

7. Fill with the broccoli-egg mixture and bake for another 25 minutes, or until the eggs are cooked (toothpick inserted in the center comes out clean) and the crust golden brown.

8. Serve hot in the baking dish.

POULTRY DISHES

CHICKEN GOULASH SOUP

This is a delicious recipe for that traditional Hungarian spicy and slightly piquant soup, goulash. Here we replace the traditional "bad" red meat (beef, pork, veal, or lamb) with chicken.

YIELD: **6** SERVINGS

Olive oil spray

2 medium white onions, finely chopped

8 ounces skinless, boneless chicken breast,
cut into $1/_2$-inch cubes

2 cups tomato sauce, or homemade Tomato Sauce Provençale
(see page 134)

2 cups chicken broth or chicken stock

1 large red bell pepper, seeded and chopped

1 teaspoon paprika powder, or more to taste

Salt, to taste

Freshly ground black pepper, to taste

1. Spray a large saucepan with the olive oil and sauté the onion over medium heat until soft and translucent, but not brown.

2. Add the chicken cubes and sauté for a few minutes, turning occasionally until golden brown.

3. Add the tomato sauce, chicken broth, and bell pepper. Season with paprika powder, salt, and pepper to taste.

4. Simmer over medium heat for about 30 minutes, or until the chicken is tender.

5. Serve immediately, or for best flavor, reheat and serve the next day.

PALEO MOUSSAKA

This Greek dish is usually made with lamb. All we need to do is substitute the meat with a better fatty acid profile meat, such as turkey (or any other fowl or wild game).

YIELD: **6** SERVINGS

3 pounds eggplant, sliced lengthways into $1/4$-inch-thick slices

2 tablespoons olive oil

$1^1/4$ pounds ground lean turkey breast (or other conforming meat)

Salt, to taste

Freshly ground black pepper, to taste

2 jars (14 ounces each) ready-made conforming marinara sauce

Tabasco sauce, to taste

Olive oil spray

1. Preheat the oven to 340°F (170°C).

2. Steam the eggplant slices for 10–15 minutes or until cooked. Separate them into three batches. Set aside.

3. Heat the oil in a large, non-stick frying pan and sauté the ground turkey over medium-high heat, taking care to crumble it with a fork during the cooking process. The turkey meat should be golden brown. Salt and pepper to taste.

3. Add the marinara sauce to the turkey and heat through. Season with the Tabasco sauce to taste.

4. Spray a large (at least 9-inch, and preferably square), table-ready baking dish with olive oil. Cover the bottom with the first batch of eggplant slices. Salt and pepper to taste.

5. Take half of the turkey and marinara mixture and spread it over the first eggplant layer. Place the second batch of eggplant in the next layer. Salt and pepper to taste.

6. Spread the remaining turkey and marinara mixture over the eggplant slices. Place the third batch of eggplant slices in a final layer to cover the whole dish. Salt and pepper to taste.

7. Bake for 10 to 15 minutes. Serve hot.

SEAFOOD AND MEAT DISHES

SALMON STEAKS WITH CAPERS

This is the classic baked salmon, rich in fish oils, but spiced up with capers and French mustard.

Yield: 2 servings

2 salmon steaks (about 5–6 ounces each)

Olive oil spray

2 teaspoons Dijon mustard

1 tablespoon olive oil

2 cloves garlic, crushed

2 tablespoons slivered almonds

1 tablespoon capers, drained

1. Preheat the oven to 340°F (170°C).

2. Rinse the salmon steaks under running water. Drain and pat dry with a paper towel.

3. Spray a medium-size baking dish with the olive oil and lay out the salmon steaks on the bottom, skin-side down.

4. Combine the mustard, olive oil, and garlic in a small mixing bowl. Coat the tops of the steaks with the mixture.

5. Bake for about 12 to 15 minutes, or until the fish can be easily flaked with a fork.

6. Meanwhile, spray a small frying pan with the oil and briefly sauté the slivered almonds. Mix in the capers and sauté over medium heat for two minutes.

7. Cover the top of the steaks with a layer of the almond-caper mixture and serve immediately.

HUNTER'S STEW

This recipe is a classic way of preparing hunted meats. It uses the technique of marinating, or soaking the meat in a flavorful liquid to tenderize the meat and enrich its flavor. Here we use venison, but you can try this recipe with other game meat, too, such as bison, wild boar, or elk.

Yield: 8 servings

Marinade

$1/2$ bottle (about $1 1/2$ cups) dry red wine

1 onion, sliced

3 garlic cloves, sliced

1 teaspoon peppercorns

1 tablespoon cinnamon bark pieces

3 bay leaves

3 sprigs fresh oregano or thyme,
or 2 teaspoons dried herbs

Stew

2 pounds venison meat, cut into 1-inch cubes

2 tablespoons olive oil, divided

1 pound onions, sliced

5 cloves garlic, crushed

2 tablespoons tomato paste

1 pound green bell peppers, seeded and sliced

2 pounds zucchini, sliced

$1/2$ pound white cabbage, sliced

Salt, to taste

Freshly ground black pepper, to taste

2 teaspoons Italian seasoning

1 teaspoon ground coriander

1 teaspoon ground cumin

Tabasco sauce, to taste

1. Combine all marinade ingredients in a medium-size dish. Add the meat and leave to marinate, covered with a lid or foil, for at least 24 hours and up to 2 days in the refrigerator (the meat should be covered by the marinade—if not, turn the meat from time to time).

2. On the day you cook the meat, drain it in a colander, but collect the liquid and keep the onion and garlic apart. Set aside.

3. Heat 1 tablespoon of the oil in a large saucepan. Add the drained venison and sauté over medium-high heat until golden brown on both sides. Set aside on a plate and cover.

4. Add the remaining tablespoon of oil to the pan and sauté the onion until it is soft and translucent, but not brown.

5. Add the garlic and sauté for 2 minutes.

6. Mix in the tomato paste and coat the onion.

7. Add the leftover marinated onion and garlic, together with the green bell peppers. Sauté for 5 minutes.

8. Mix in the zucchini and the cabbage.

9. Season with salt and pepper to taste. Add the Italian seasoning, the coriander, the cumin, and the Tabasco sauce to taste.

10. Add the reserved marinade liquid as needed to moisten the vegetables.

11. Cook covered, until the veggies are half-cooked but still very crunchy.

12. Add the reserved venison meat. Simmer all together for about 15 minutes, or more if needed to cook the meat as desired. Serve hot.

SARDINE SOUFFLÉ ON TOAST

*An interesting and sophisticated variant
on traditional sardines on toast.*

YIELD: **4** SLICES

4-ounce can sardines, in olive oil or tomato sauce

4 slices Almond Flour Bread (see page 128)

1 egg white, omega-3

Ground black pepper, to taste

Ground paprika, to taste

1. Drain the sardines and remove the backbones. Crush sardines with a fork. Set aside.

2. In a toaster, lightly toast 4 slices of bread.

3. Beat the egg white with an electric hand-mixer in a small mixing bowl until it reaches a stiff consistency.

4. Mix the egg white carefully into the sardines. Add pepper to taste.

5. Spread the sardine mix uniformly on the toasted bread slices, making sure to cover the edges.

6. Arrange slices on the oven's grilling shelf.

7. Grill under a medium heat until the top is golden brown (about 5 to 10 minutes).

8. Sprinkle with ground paprika to taste and serve immediately.

DESSERTS

CHOCOLATE DELIGHT

This recipe provides an impressive and delicious chocolate torte. Because the dish is fundamentally energy-dense, you should limit yourself to just one serving at a sitting. Try serving with raspberry coulis for a fruity contrast.

YIELD: 10-INCH TORTE

2 bars ($3^1/_2$ ounces each) dark chocolate (minimum of 75 percent cocoa solids), broken into small pieces

$^3/_4$ cup almond milk

1 tablespoon dark rum

4 omega-3 eggs

2 tablespoons olive oil

1 teaspoon orange extract

3 tablespoons sugar-free orange marmalade

3 tablespoons almond flour

Olive oil spray

1. Preheat the oven to 340°F (170°C).

2. Put chocolate pieces in a medium-size microwave-proof bowl. Add the almond milk.

3. Melt the mixture at half-power (about 300 watts) in a microwave oven for 3 to 4 minutes. Check and stir after every minute. The chocolate should be melted, but avoid overheating. Mix in the rum and set aside.

4. Beat the eggs in a medium-size mixing bowl with an electric hand mixer. Blend in the olive oil, orange extract, orange marmalade, and almond flour.

5. Add the chocolate mixture to the eggs, and blend to a smooth consistency.

6. Spray a round 10-inch table-ready baking dish with the olive oil. Slowly pour the mixture into it.

7. Bake for about 15 minutes. The center of this chocolate delight should still be slightly moist. Allow to cool before serving.

MARBLE RING CAKE

*This recipe makes a wonderful, fully-conforming marble cake
that will delight children and adults alike.*

YIELD: 8- OR 9-INCH CAKE

5 omega-3 eggs

6 tablespoons xylitol, or to taste, divided

4 tablespoons olive oil, divided

1 teaspoon baking powder

2 cups almond flour

2 teaspoons vanilla extract

$1/2$ cup cocoa powder

1 tablespoon dark rum

$1/4$ cup almond milk (or more, if needed)

Olive oil spray

1. Preheat the oven to 340°F (170°C).

2. In a medium-size mixing bowl, beat the eggs with an electric hand mixer. Blend in 4 tablespoons of xylitol, 3 tablespoons of olive oil, and the baking powder. Add the almond flour and blend to obtain a smooth paste.

3. Divide the batter into two equal portions, and place in two separate mixing bowls.

4. In one bowl, blend in the vanilla extract. This will be the "light-colored batter."

5. In the second portion, blend in the remaining 2 tablespoons xylitol, the remaining 1 tablespoon olive oil, the cocoa powder, the rum, and the almond milk, adding more milk if the batter is too thick. This will be the "dark-colored batter."

6. Spray an 8- or 9-inch ring cake mold with the olive oil. Pour light colored and dark colored batter layers randomly into the mold. You can play with the proportions of light and dark layers to make an interesting "marbling."

7. Bake for about 30 minutes, or until the center of the cake is firm (not moist). Allow to cool in fridge before unmolding and serving.

Fluffy Version:

1. To make a fluffier version of the cake, separate the egg yolks and the egg whites into two medium-size mixing bowls.

2. Beat the egg yolks with 4 tablespoons of xylitol, 3 tablespoons of olive oil, the baking powder, and the almond flour. Set aside.

3. With an electric hand mixer, beat the egg whites to a stiff consistency.

4. Fold the egg whites carefully into the egg yolk mixture.

5. Split into two equal portions and continue from step 3 of the directions on page 144.

STRAWBERRY ICE CREAM

When I had finished refining this recipe, it came out more like a sorbet, with little fat or cream. It is absolutely delicious and leaves a clean taste on the palate. Everybody loves these delicious and safe ice cream recipes, since they are made without dairy and sugar, which are the usual bad ingredients in conventional ice creams.

YIELD: **14** SERVINGS

2 pounds frozen strawberries, defrosted

1 cup Thai-style coconut milk

10 tablespoons sugar-free strawberry jam

2 tablespoons vanilla extract

1 teaspoon xanthan gum

4–5 tablespoons xylitol, to taste

1. Place strawberries in a food processor and purée until smooth.

2. Mix in the coconut milk, strawberry jam, vanilla extract, and xanthan gum. Sweeten with xylitol to taste and blend.

3. Place the mixture in an ice cream maker and follow the manufacturer's instructions. If you do not have an ice cream maker, place the mixture in a bowl, which you then place in the freezer. From time to time, you will need to fold the frozen edges in towards the middle to lighten the mixture. Do this after 1 hour, once more after the second hour, and then every 30 minutes for the next 2 hours. Serve immediately.

Resources

I passionately believe in the insights contained in this work. My driving motivation is to stimulate everyone, no matter your origins and background, to improve your lives. I hope that this book has inspired and encouraged you to know more. The following list is a reservoir of resources I have curated to help you put the Paleo principles into practice.

WEBSITES

The Bond Effect Website • www.thebondeffect.com
Your first port of call should be my website, www.TheBondEffect.com. There you will find online support, speaking engagements, breaking news, updates, hints and tips, and much more. In addition, you can acquire access to many other support materials.

Glycemic Index and Glycemic Load • www.glycemicindex.com
A prime feature of the Savanna Model is to eat a low-glycemic diet. Scientists have tested a great many foods (most of them processed) and this website, compiled by Jennie Brand-Miller at Sydney University, contains a compendium of the test results. However, many of the tests need to be interpreted; we do not agree with the *interpretation* that Brand-Miller puts on the tests. With these caveats, the raw data is a valuable resource.

National Institutes of Health (NIH) • www.nih.gov
The NIH is a part of the U.S. Department of Health and Human Services and is the primary federal agency for conducting and supporting medical research. Its results are less likely to be tainted by commercial pressures than from other sources.

United States Department of Agriculture (USDA) • www.usda.gov
The USDA is the home of the infamous food pyramids/plates and the Dietary Guidelines for Americans. These jostle for visibility among the USDA's advice to farmers about subsidies for sugar production and how to persuade unwilling

Japanese to import American hormone-treated beef. The USDA's nutrition database at www.nal.usda.gov is a useful compendium of the composition of a wide variety of foods. Most of the foods are processed and proprietary brands, but this is still invaluable for generic foodstuffs as well.

United States Food and Drug Administration (FDA) • www.fda.gov
Here you can follow how the FDA tries to hold the line against the food industry's pressure to approve all kinds of unsuitable products for human consumption and make health claims to boot.

RECOMMENDED READING

I have included all the relevant books in the list of references, but here is a selection of the primary sources readily accessible to the interested reader.

The Blank Slate: The Modern Denial of Human Nature by Steven Pinker (New York: Penguin, 2003). Pinker, with surgical precision, slices away the myth of the "noble savage" to replace it with a wide-ranging exposé of the deep undercurrents driving human behavior.

Deadly Harvest by Geoff Bond (Garden City Park, NY: Square One Publishers, 2007). This is my Bible to current thinking on Evolutionary Lifestyle Anthropology. It contains all the background and supporting information to back up the assertions and simplifications in this guide.

Demonic Males: Apes and the Origins of Human Violence by Richard Wrangham and Dale Peterson (Boston: Houghton Mifflin, 1996). The authors dispel the notion that human males are "depraved because they are deprived." Here, they compare the behavior of human foragers, gorillas, and the most violent of all, the chimpanzee. If we are to channel violence, war, and hatred, we have to understand how these forces came about in our evolutionary past.

Fiji's Times: History of Fiji by Kim Gravelle (Suva, Fiji: Fiji Times, 1988). A review of the bloodthirsty history of Fiji before and during Western contact. An insight into the natural history of this fishing and gardening, yet warlike, society that made cannibalism an integral part of its dietary habits.

Gorillas in the Mist by Dian Fossey (Boston: Houghton Mifflin, 1983). A riveting account of the first studies in the wild on our next closest cousin, the gorilla.

Guns, Germs, and Steel: The Fates of Human Societies by Jared Diamond (New York: W.W. Norton, 1999). This broad sweep of human history explains how, where, and why agriculture developed over the last 13,000 years. It describes the types of new plants and creatures that farmers domesticated and how their new lifestyle changed the fortunes of their societies.

The Hadza Hunter-Gatherers of Tanzania by Frank W. Marlowe (Oakland, CA: University of California Press, 2010). Frank Marlowe is a long-time researcher of one of the last hunter-gatherer populations of the world, the Hadza. He provides a meticulously documented, rigorous, and shrewd analysis of his studies over many years since the 1990s. It, too, is wide-ranging, covering—amongst other things—habitat, social organization, beliefs and practices, foraging, parenting, cooperation, and food sharing.

The Hero with a Thousand Faces by Joseph Campbell. (Novato, CA: New World Library, 2008). Joseph Campbell was an extraordinary authority on comparative mythology. His deep insights into the stories, beliefs, and religions worldwide are incredibly illuminating. All such mythology distills itself down to a few grand themes to be found in every culture—including hunter-gatherers. Indeed, George Lucas consulted Joseph Campbell when developing his *Star Wars* epic. Campbell has authored a huge compendium of works, and *The Hero* is a useful digest of the main principles. It fruitfully illuminates other hunter-gatherer studies of spirituality and belief.

In the Shadow of Man by Jane Goodall (Boston: Houghton Mifflin, 1988). A classic account of the first studies in the wild on our closest cousin, the chimpanzee. Includes many insights into how they lived their lives and fed themselves.

Kalahari Hunter-Gatherers: Studies of the !Kung San and Their Neighbors by Richard Lee and Irven DeVore, editors (Cambridge, MA: Harvard University Press, 1976). A classic of hunter-gatherer research carried out for over fifteen years from 1963 onwards at a time when there were still a few !Kung San bands living the traditional way. The studies are wide-ranging, covering ecology and social change, population and health, childhood, and behavior and belief.

The Lost World of the Kalahari by Laurens van der Post (New York: Harcourt Brace & Company, 1986). Written by the South African explorer and guru to Prince Charles, this is an inspiring account of van der Post's expeditions in the 1950s to discover the lives and fate of the disappearing San Bushmen. Contains fascinating information on their hunter-gatherer feeding habits.

The Natural World of the California Indians by Robert Fleming Heizer and Albert B. Elasser (Berkeley, CA: University of California Press, 1981). Most American Indian tribes were hunter-gatherers until the arrival of Europeans. This book describes the people, how they lived, what they manufactured, and in some cases what they thought, before their traditional aboriginal way of life was destroyed.

Paleo Harvest: Healthy Cooking with The Bond Girl by Nicole Bond. (London: Bond Effect Publications, 2015). This is my wife Nicole's essential handmaiden to everyone living the Bond Effect way. It contains interesting, tasty, and practical recipes that fit in with the Bond Effect precepts. Available at www.Paleo-Harvest.com.

The Selfish Gene by Richard Dawkins (Oxford: Oxford University Press, 1989). This classic work, for the first time, shifted our focus to the level of the gene. Its great insight was to understand that the fundamental force driving the behavior of all living things is that of gene success. In the words of the author: "We are survival machines, robot vehicles blindly programmed to preserve the selfish molecules known as genes."

Triumph of the Nomads: A History of Ancient Australia by Geoffrey Blainey (South Melbourne, Australia: Macmillan, 1982). The Australian Aboriginals were the last major group of hunter-gatherers to come into contact with the West. As such, we have many explorers' accounts of their ancient way of life. Blainey has drawn this knowledge together in a readable and informative book.

Vaka: Saga of a Polynesian Canoe by Thomas R.A.H. Davis (Auckland, New Zealand: Polynesian Press, 1992). A precious and rare account by the royal chief of the Cook Islands, relating how the seafaring and gardening societies of Polynesia lived their lives before Western contact.

OTHER RESOURCES

The Bond Briefing Newsletter

Everyone serious about adopting the Savanna Model will find my monthly newsletter an indispensable aid to keep focused on the essentials. Editors of mainstream food magazines cannot afford to upset their advertisers, so their editorial matter is at best bland, uncontroversial, and meaningless. The Bond Briefing takes no advertising and so it is free to give an honest, straight-from-the-shoulder, Bond Effect viewpoint. It typically contains packed pages of hints, tips, health updates, food/disease connections, readers' questions and answers, recipes, the Bond Effect view of breaking news, survival skills (marketing campaigns debunked), and much more. Subscribe at www.TheBondEffect.com.

Consumer Lobbies

Center for Science in the Public Interest • www.cspinet.org

Physicians' Committee for Responsible Medicine • www.pcrm.org
Many groups are fighting the tidal wave of food industry propaganda. These two lobbies, although they occasionally take positions on some issues that we do not agree with, cast a light on the dark and grubby corners that the food industry wants to keep under wraps.

References

Introduction

1. Dong, Xiao, et al. "Evidence for a limit to human lifespan." *Nature* 538 (2016):257–259.

2. The United Nations Statistics Division. "Life expectancy at specified ages for each sex, 2015. http://unstats.un.org/unsd/demographic/products/dyb/dyb2014/Table21.pdf. Accessed 21 Dec. 2016.

Chapter 1   Origin and Main Features

1. Truswell, S., and J. Hansen. "Medical Research Among the !Kung." *Kalahari Hunter-Gatherers: Studies of the !Kung San and Their Neighbors*, ed. Richard B. Lee and Irven DeVore. Cambridge, MA: Harvard University Press, 1976.

2. Jarvis, JF, and H.G. van Heerden. "The Acuity of Hearing in the Kalahari Bushmen. A pilot survey." *Journal of Laryngology and Otology*, vol. 81, 1967: 63.

3. Burkitt, Denis. *Don't forget fibre in your diet: to help avoid many of our commonest diseases*. London: Martin Dunitz Ltd., 1979.

4. Burkitt, DP, et al. "Effect of dietary fibre on stools and the transit-times, and its role in the causation of disease." *Lancet*, vol. 2, no. 7792, 1972: 1408–1412.

5.Holt, SH, et al. "An insulin index of foods: the insulin demand generated by 1000-kJ portions of common foods." *The American Journal of Clinical Nutrition*, vol. 66, no. 5, 1997:1264–1276.

6. Oldenhove, G, et al. "Decrease of Foxp3+ Treg cell number and acquisition of effector cell phenotype during lethal infection." *Immunity*, vol. 31, no. 5, 2009: 772–786.

7. Ivanov II, et al. "Specific microbiota direct the differentiation of IL-17-producing T-helper cells in the mucosa of the small intestine." *Cell Host & Microbe*, vol. 4, no. 4, 2008: 337–349.

8. Wen, Li, et al. "Innate immunity and intestinal microbiota in the development of Type 1 diabetes." *Nature*, vol. 455, 2008: 1109–1113.

9. Jangi, Sushrut, et al. "Alterations of the human gut microbiome in multiple sclerosis." *Nature Communications*, vol. 7, 2016. DOI: 10.1038/ncomms12015.

10. Cryan, JF, et al. "Gut microbiome: a key regulator of neurodevelopment and behaviour." Second Congress of the European Academy of Neurology (EAN), Copenhagen, 2016.

11. Krishnamoorthy, G. "Microbiota and CNS autoimmunity (Multiple Sclerosis)." Second Congress of the European Academy of Neurology (EAN), Copenhagen, 2016.

12. Oury, F, and G Karsenty. "Intestinal serotonin and regulation of bone mass." *Med Sci (Paris)*, vol. 25, no. 5, 2009: 445–446.

13. Baldock, P, et al. "Neuropeptide Y Knockout Mice Reveal a Central Role of NPY in the Coordination of Bone Mass to Body Weight." *PLoS One*, vol. 4, no. 12, 2009.

14. Klumpp, DJ, and CN Rudick. "Summation model of pelvic pain in interstitial cystitis." *Natural Clinical Practice Urology*, vol. 5, no. 9, 2008: 494–500.

15. Abrahamsson, TR, et al. "Low diversity of the gut microbiota in infants with atopic eczema." *Journal of Allergy and Clinical Immunology*, vol. 129, no. 2, 2012: 434–440.

16. Bailey, MT, et al. "Exposure to a social stressor alters the structure of the intestinal microbiota: Implications for stressor-induced immuno-modulation?" *Brain, behavior, and immunity*, vol. 25, no. 3, 2011: 397–407.

17. Lepage, Patricia. "Microbiota and the gut-brain axis." Second Congress of the European Academy of Neurology (EAN), Copenhagen, 2016.

18. Clarke, G, et al. "The microbiome-gut-brain axis during early life regulates the hippocampal serotonergic system in a sex-dependent manner." *Molecular Psychiatry*, vol. 18, no. 6, 2013: 666–673.

19. Diaz Heijtz, R, et al. "Normal gut microbiota modulates brain development and behavior." *Proceedings of the National Academy of Sciences USA*, vol. 108, no. 7, 2011: 3047–3052.

20. Kavli Foundation. www.kavlifoundation.org. Accessed 8 January 2015.

21. Magnusson, KR, et al. "Relationships between diet-related changes in the gut microbiome and cognitive flexibility." *Neuroscience*, vol. 300, 2015: 128–140.

22. Christian, L, et al. "Gut microbiome composition is associated with temperament during early childhood." *Brain, behavior, and immunity*, vol. 45, 2015: 118–127.

23. Mardinoglu, A, et al. "The gut microbiota modulates host amino acid and glutathione metabolism in mice." *Molecular Systems Biology*, vol. 11, no. 10, 2015: 834.

24. Zhernakova, A, et al. "Population-based meta-genomics analysis reveals markers for gut microbiome composition and diversity." *Science* vol. 352, no. 6285, 2016: 565–569.

25. Falony, G, et al. "Population-level analysis of gut microbiome variation." *Science* vol. 352, no. 6285, 2016.

26. Turnbaugh, PJ, et al. "An obesity-associated gut microbiome with increased capacity for energy harvest." *Nature* vol. 444, 2006: 1027–1031.

27. Horai, R, et al. "Microbiota-Dependent Activation of an Auto-reactive T Cell Receptor Provokes Autoimmunity." *Immunity*, vol. 43, no. 2, 2015: 343–353.

Chapter 2 Living the Way Nature Intended

1. Calhoun, John. "Population Density and Social Pathology." *Calif Med*, vol. 113, no. 5, 1970: 54.

2. Binder, M, and A Coad. "Life satisfaction and self-employment: a matching approach." *Small Business Economics*, vol. 40, no. 4, 2013: 1009–1033.

3. Hawkes, K, et al. "Grandmothering, menopause, and the evolution of human life histories." *Proceedings of the National Academy of Science USA*, vol. 95, 1998: 1336–1339.

4. Bond, Geoff. *Deadly Harvest*. Garden City Park, NY: Square One Publishers, 2007. pp. 269.

5. Shah, I, et al. "Low 25OH Vitamin D2 Levels Found in Untreated Alzheimer's Patients." *Current Alzheimer's Research*, vol. 9, no. 9, 2012: 1069–1076.

6. Wehr, T.A., et al. "A Circadian Signal of Change of Season in Patients with Seasonal Affective Disorder." *Archives of General Psychiatry*, vol. 58, no. 12, 2001: 1108–1114.

7. Ramagopalan, SV, et al. "Expression of the Multiple Sclerosis-Associated MHC Class II Allele HLA-DRB1*1501 Is Regulated by Vitamin D." *PLoS Genetics*, vol 5., no. 2, 2009: e1000369

8. Munger, K.L., et al. "Vitamin D Intake and Incidence of Multiple Sclerosis." *Neurology* vol. 62, no. 1, 2004: 60–65.

9. Chiu, K.C., et. al. "Hypovitaminosis D is Associated with Insulin Resistance and Beta Cell Dysfunction." *American Journal of Clinical Nutrition*, vol. 79, no. 5, 2004: 820–825.

10. John, E.M., et al. "Vitamin D and Breast Cancer Risk: The NHANES I Epidemiologic Follow-up Study, 1971–1975 to 1992. National Health and Nutrition Examination Survey." *Cancer Epidemiology, Biomarkers and Prevention*, vol. 8, no. 5, 1999: 399–406.

11. Grant, WB. "An Estimate of Premature Cancer Mortality in the U.S. Due to Inadequate Doses of Solar Ultraviolet-B Radiation." *Cancer* vol. 94, no. 6, 2002: 1867–1875.

12. John, EM, et al. "Sun Exposure, Vitamin D Receptor Gene Polymorphisms, and Risk of Advanced Prostate Cancer." *Cancer Research* vol. 65, no. 12, 2005: 5470–5479.

13. Garland, C.F., et al. "Serum 25-hydroxyvitamin D and Colon Cancer: Eight-year Prospective Study." *Lancet* vol. 2, no. 8673, 1989: 1176–1178.

14. Berwick, M., et al. "Sun Exposure and Mortality From Melanoma." *Journal of the National Cancer Institute* 97:3 (2005): 195–199.

15. Smedby, K.E., H. Hjalgrim, M. Melbye, et al. "Ultraviolet Radiation Exposure and Risk of Malignant Lymphomas." *Journal of the National Cancer Institute* 97:3 (2005): 199–209.

16. Chevalier, C, et al. "Gut Microbiota Orchestrates Energy Homeostasis during Cold." *Cell*, vol. 163, no. 6, 2015.

17. Rostand, S.G. "Ultraviolet Light May Contribute to Geographic and Racial Blood Pressure Differences." *Hypertension* vol. 30, no. 2 Part 1, 1997: 150–156.

18. Cantorna, M.T., et al. "1,25-dihydroxycholecalciferol Prevents and Ameliorates Symptoms of Experimental Murine Inflammatory Bowel Disease." *Journal of Nutrition*, vol. 130, no. 11, 2000: 2648–2652.

19. Shuster, Sam. "Is sun exposure a major cause of melanoma? No." *BMJ* vol. 337, 2008:a764.

20. Taksler, GB, et al. "Vitamin D deficiency in minority populations." *Public Health Nutrition*, vol. 18, no. 3, 2015: 379–391.

— Grant, WB, and AN Peiris. "Possible role of serum 25-hydroxyvitamin D in black-white health disparities in the United States." *Journal of the American Medical Directors Association*, vol. 11, no. 9, 2010: 617–628.

21. Yetish, G, et al. "Natural Sleep and Its Seasonal Variations in Three Pre-industrial Societies." *Current Biology,* vol. 25, no. 21, 2015: 2862–2868.

22. Reid, KJ, et al. "Timing and Intensity of Light Correlate with Body Weight in Adults." *PLoS One,* vol. 9, no. 4, 2014: e92251.

23. Foster, Russell. "Why Do We Sleep?" *TED Global 2013: Exquisite Enigmatic Us,* 11 June 2013, Edinburgh International Conference Center, Scotland. TED Talk. https://www.ted.com/talks/russell_foster_why_do_we_sleep

24. Harvard Medical School, Division of Sleep Medicine. "Sleep, Learning, and Memory." 18 Dec. 2007. http://healthysleep.med.harvard.edu/healthy/matters/benefits-of-sleep/learning-memory

25. Ackermann, K, et al. "Diurnal rhythms in blood cell populations and the effect of acute sleep deprivation in healthy young men." *Sleep,* vol. 35, no. 7, 2012: 933–940.

26. Caruso, CC. "Negative Impacts of Shiftwork and Long Work Hours." *Rehabil Nurs* vol. 39, no. 1, 2014: 16–25.

27. National Sleep Foundation. "Sleep Longer to Lower Blood Glucose Levels." https://sleepfoundation.org/excessivesleepiness/content/sleep-longer-lower-blood-glucose-levels

28. Taheri, S, et al. "Short sleep duration is associated with reduced leptin, elevated ghrelin, and increase body mass index." *PLoS Med,* vol. 1, no. 3, 2004: e62.

29. Xie, L, et al. "Sleep Drives Metabolite Clearance from the Adult Brain." *Science,* vol. 342, no. 6156, 2013: 373–377.

30. Smith, SM, and M Heer. "Calcium and bone metabolism during space flight." *Nutrition* vol. 18, no. 10, 2002: 849–852.

Chapter 3 How Did It Go Wrong?

1. Giacco, R, et al. "Characteristics of some wheat-based foods of the Italian diet in relation to their influence on postprandial glucose metabolism in patients with type 2 diabetes." *British Journal of Nutrition,* vol. 85, no. 1, 2001: 33–40.

— Lee, BM, and TM Wolever. "Effect of glucose, sucrose and fructose on plasma glucose and insulin responses in normal humans: comparison with white bread." *European Journal of Clinical Nutrition* vol. 52, no. 12, 1998: 924–928.

— The University of Sydney. *Glycemic Index database.* http://www.glycemicindex.com. Accessed 18 January 2017.

2. de Punder, K, and L Pruimboom. "The dietary intake of wheat and other cereal grains and their role in inflammation." *Nutrients* vol. 5, no. 3, 2013: 771–787.

3. Podolak, I, et al. "Saponins as cytotoxic agents: a review." *Phytochemistry Reviews* vol. 9, no. 3, 2010: 425–474.

4. Delvecchio, M, et al. "Anti-pituitary antibodies in children with newly diagnosed celiac disease: a novel finding contributing to linear-growth impairment." *American Journal of Gastroenterology* vol. 105, no. 3, 2010: 691–696.

5. Fish, BC, and LU Thompson. "Lectin-tannin interactions and their influence on pancreatic amylase activity and starch digestibility." *Journal of Agricultural and Food Chemistry,* vol. 39, no. 4, 1991: 727–731.

6. Shahidi, F. "Beneficial health effects and drawbacks of antinutrients and phytochemicals in foods: an overview." In *ACS Symposium Series*, American Chemical Society, Washington, DC, 1997: 1–9.

7. Harvard Medical School, Harvard Health Publications. "Glycemic index and glycemic load for 100+ foods." —Harvard Medical School. 2015 Aug. 27. http://www.health.harvard.edu/diseases-and-conditions/glycemic_index_and_glycemic_load_for_100_foods

8. "Potato Nutritional Summary: Micronutrient removal." *Yara*. Accessed 18 January 2017. http://www.yara.us/agriculture/crops/potato/key-facts/nutritional-summary/

9. Cantwell, Marita. "A review of important facts about potato glycoalkaloids." *Perishables Handling Newsletter* no. 87, 1996: 26–27. http://ucce.ucdavis.edu/files/datastore/234-182.pdf

10. Shepherd, Peter. "Balancing acid/alkaline foods." *Trans4mind*. Accessed 18 January 2017. https://trans4mind.com/nutrition/pH.html

11. Bond, Geoff. *Deadly Harvest*. Garden City Park, NY: Square One Publishers, 2007. pp. 17.

12. Crittenden, A. "The importance of honey consumption in human evolution." *Food and Foodways*, vol. 19, no. 4, 2011: 257–273.

13. Allsop, KA, and JB Miller. "Honey revisited: a reappraisal of honey in pre-industrial diets." *British Journal of Nutrition*, vol. 75, no. 4, 1996: 513–520.

14. United States Department of Agriculture, Economic Research Service. "Sugar and Sweeteners Yearbook Tables." 19 Dec 2016. https://www.ers.usda.gov/data-products/sugar-and-sweeteners-yearbook-tables/

— Johnson, RJ, et al. "Potential role of sugar (fructose) in the epidemic of hypertension, obesity and the metabolic syndrome, diabetes, kidney disease, and cardiovascular disease." *American Journal of Clinical Nutrition*, vol. 86, no. 4, 2007: 899–906.

— Yudkin, J. "Sugar and disease." *Nature* vol. 239, 1972: 197–199.

15. Gilani, GS, et al. "Effects of antinutritional factors on protein digestibility and amino acid availability in foods." *Journal of AOAC International* vol. 88, no. 3, 2005; 967–987.

16. Newbold, RR, et al. "Uterine adenocarcinoma in mice treated neonatally with genistein." *Cancer Research* vol. 61, no. 11, 2001: 4325–4328.

17. Allred, CD, et al. "Dietary genistin stimulates growth of estrogen-dependent breast cancer tumors similar to that observed with genistein." *Carcinogenesis* vol. 22, no. 10, 2001: 1667–1673.

—Ju, YH, et al. "Physiological concentrations of dietary genistein dose-dependently stimulate growth of estrogen-dependent human breast cancer (mcf-7) tumors implanted in athymic nude mice." *The Journal of Nutrition* vol. 131, no. 11, 2001: 2957–2962.

—Allred, CD, et al. "Soy diets containing varying amounts of genistein stimulate growth of estrogen-dependent (mcf-7) tumors in a dose-dependent manner." *Cancer Research* vol. 61, no. 13, 2001: 5045–5050.

18. Divi, RL, et al. "Anti-thyroid isoflavones from soybean: isolation, characterization, and mechanisms of action." *Biochemical Pharmacology* vol. 54, no. 10, 1997: 1087–1096.

19. White, LR, et al. "Brain aging and midlife tofu consumption." *Journal of American College of Nutrition* vol. 19, no. 2, 2000: 242–255.

20. Sharom, FJ, et al. "Inhibition of lymphocyte 5'-nucleotidase by lectins: effects of lectin specifity and cross-linking ability." *Biochemistry and Cell Biology,* vol. 66, no. 7, 1988: 715–723.

21. Foucard, T, and I Malmheden Yman. "A study on severe food reactions in Sweden—is soy protein an underestimated cause of food anaphylaxis?" *Allergy* vol. 54, no. 3, 1999: 261–265.

— Tsuji, H, et al. "Allergens in major crops." *Nutrition Research* vol. 21, no. 6, 2001: 925–934.

22. Centers for Disease Control (CDC). "Table 56 (page 1 of 2). Mean macronutrient intake among adults aged 20 and over, by sex and age: United States, selected years 1988–1994 through 2009–2012." Accessed 18 Jan 2017. https://www.cdc.gov/nchs/data/hus/hus15.pdf#222

23. Blasbalg, TL, et al. "Changes in consumption of omega-3 and omega-6 fatty acids in the United States during the 20th century." *The American Journal of Clinical Nutrition,* vol. 93, no. 5, 2011: 950–962.

24. Barnard, ND. "Trends in food availability, 1909–2007." *The American Journal of Clinical Nutrition,* vol. 91, no. 5, 2010: 1530S–1536S.

25. World Health Organization (WHO) and Food and Agriculture Organization of the United Nations (FAO). "Diet, Nutrition, and the Prevention of Chronic Diseases." *WHO Technical Report Series,* 2003.

26. Crawford, MA. "Fatty acid ratios in free-living and domestic animals. Possible implications for atheroma." *Lancet* vol. 1, no. 7556, 1968: 1329–1333.

27. French, P, et al. "Fatty acid composition, including conjugated linoleic acid, of intramuscular fat from steers offered grazed grass, grass silage, or concentrate-based diets." *Journal of Animal Science* vol. 78, no. 11, 2000. 2849–2855.

28. Crawford, MA. "Food selection under natural conditions and the possible relationship to heart disease in man." *The Proceedings of the Nutrition Society,* vol. 27, no. 2, 1968: 163–172.

29. Hoppe, C, et al. "Differential effects of casein versus whey on fasting plasma levels of insulin, IGF-1 and IGF-1/IGFBP-3: results from a randomized 7-day supplementation study in prepubertal boys." *European Journal of Clinical Nutrition* vol. 63, 2009: 1076–1083.

30. Duarte, SD, et al. "Are the high hip fracture rates among Norwegian women explained by impaired bone material properties?" *Journal of Bone and Mineral Research,* vol. 30, no. 10, 2015: 1784–1789.

31. Feskanich, D, et al. "Milk, dietary calcium, and bone fractures in women: a 12-year prospective study." *American Journal of Public Health* vol. 87, no. 6, 1997: 992–997.

32. Truswell, S., and J. Hansen. "Medical Research Among the !Kung." *Kalahari Hunter-Gatherers: Studies of the !Kung San and Their Neighbors,* ed. Richard B. Lee and Irven DeVore. Cambridge, MA: Harvard University Press, 1976.

33.Nilas, L. "Calcium intake and osteoporosis." *World Review of Nutrition and Dietetics* vol. 73, 1993: 1–26.

34. Srivatsa, SS, et al. "Increased cellular expression of matrix proteins that regulate mineralization is associated with calcification of native human and porcine xenograft bioprosthetic heart valves." *Journal of Clinical Investigation* vol. 99, no. 5, 1997: 996–1009.

35. Jackson, RD, et al. "Calcium plus vitamin D supplementation and the risk of fractures." *The New England Journal of Medicine* vol. 354, no. 7, 2006: 669–683.

36. Chan, JM, et al. "Dairy products, calcium and prostate cancer risk in the Physicians' Health Study." *The American Journal of Clinical Nutrition,* vol. 74, no. 4, 2001: 549–554.

37. De Stefani, E, et al. "Fatty foods and the risk of lung cancer: a case-control study from Uruguay." *International Journal of Cancer,* vol. 71, no. 5, 1997: 760–766.

38. Grant, WB. "Milk and other dietary influences on coronary heart disease." *Alternative Medicine Review* vol. 3, no. 4, 1998: 281–294.

39. "Plant foods and atherosclerosis." *Nutrition Reviews,* vol. 35, no. 6, 1977: 148–150.

40. Ratner, D, et al. "Milk protein-free diet for nonseasonal asthma and migraine in lactase-deficient patients." *Israel Journal of Medical Sciences,* vol. 19, no. 9, 1983: 806–809.

41. Riordan, AM, et al. "Treatment of active Crohn's disease by exclusion diet: East Anglian multicentre controlled trial." *Lancet* vol. 342, no. 8880, 1993: 1131–1134.

42. Renaud, S. Personal communication, July 22, 1997.

43. Holt, SH, et al. "An insulin index of foods: the insulin demand generated by 1000-kJ portions of common foods." *The American Journal of Clinical Nutrition* vol. 66, no. 5, 1997: 1264–1276.

44. Geisel School of Medicine at Dartmouth. "Professor Finds No Scientific Evidence for Watery Urban Myth." *DMS Digest,* July/Aug 2002. http://geiselmed.dartmouth.edu/News/publications/news_digest/digest0802/myth.shtml

45. Hew-Butler, T, et al. "Statement of the 3rd International Exercise-Associated Hyponatremia Consensus Development Conference, Carlsbad, California, 2015." *British Journal of Sports Medicine,* vol. 25, no. 4, 2015: 303

46. Cohen, D. "The Truth About Sports Drinks." *BMJ,* vol. 345, 2012: 20–28. http://www.bmj.com/bmj/section-pdf/187587?path=/bmj/345/7866/Feature.full.pdf

Chapter 4 The Owner's Manual

1. Pollock, NK, et al. "Greater fructose consumption is associated with cardiometabolic risk markers and visceral adiposity in adolescents." *Journal of Nutrition,* vol. 142, no. 2, 2011: 251–257.

2. Guy, CD, et al. "Hedgehog pathway activation parallels histologic severity of injury and fibrosis in human nonalcoholic fatty liver disease." *Hepatology,* vol. 55, no. 6, 2012: 1711–1721.

3. Saad, AF, et al. "High-fructose diet in pregnancy leads to fetal programming of hypertension, insulin resistance, and obesity in adult offspring." *American Journal of Obstetrics and Gynecology,* vol. 215, no. 3, 2016: 378.e1–6.

4. Saad, AF, et al. "Maternal fructose consumption disrupts brain development of offspring in a murine model of autism spectrum disorder." *American Journal of Perinatology* vol. 33, no. 14, 2016: 1357–1364.

5. Agrawal, R, and F. Gomez-Pinilla. "'Metabolic syndrome' in the brain: deficiency in omega-3 fatty acid exacerbates dysfunctions in insulin receptor signalling and cognition." *The Journal of Physiology,* vol. 590, no. 10, 2012: 2485–2499.

6. Kavanagh, K, et al. "Dietary fructose induces endotoxemia and hepatic injury in calorically controlled primates." *American Journal of Clinical Nutrition,* vol. 98, no. 2, 2013: 349–357.

7. DiNicolantonio, JJ, et al. "Added fructose: a principal driver of type 2 diabetes mellitus and its consequences." *Mayo Clinic Proceedings,* 2015.

8. Ruff, JS, et al. "Compared to sucrose, previous consumption of fructose and glucose monosaccharides reduces survival and fitness of female mice." *The Journal of Nutrition,* vol. 145, no. 3, 2015: 434–441.

9. Rendeiro, C, et al. "Fructose decreases physical activity and increases body fat without affecting hippocampal neurogenesis and learning relative to an isocaloric glucose diet." *Scientific Reports,* vol. 5, no. 9589, 2015.

10. Mirtschink, P, et al. "HIF-driven *SF3B1* induces KHK-C to enforce fructolysis and heart disease." *Nature,* vol. 552, 2015: 444–449.

11. Agrawal, R, et al. "Dietary fructose aggravates the pathobiology of traumatic brain injury by influencing energy homeostasis and plasticity." *Journal of Cerebral Blood Flow and Metabolism,* vol. 36, no. 5, 2016: 941–953.

12. Bray, GA. "Fructose: pure, white, and deadly? Fructose, by any other name, is a health hazard." *Journal of Diabetes Science and Technology,* vol. 4, no. 4, 2010: 1003–1007.

13. Mäkinen, KK, et al. "Topical xylitol administration by parents for the promotion of oral health in infants: a caries prevention experiment at a Finnish Public Health Centre." *International Dental Journal,* vol. 63, no. 4, 2013: 210–224.

14. Teff, K. "Nutritional implications of the cephalic-phase reflexes: endocrine responses." *Appetite* vol. 34, no. 2, 2000: 206–213.

— Power, ML, and J Schulkin. "Anticipatory physiological regulation in feeding biology: cephalic phase responses." *Appetite* vol. 50, no. 2–3, 2008: 194–206.

15. Suez, J, et al. "Artificial sweeteners induce glucose intolerance by altering the gut microbiota." *Nature* vol. 514, 2014: 181–186.

16. Abou-Donia, MB, et al. "Splenda alters gut microflora and increases intestinal p-glycoprotein and cytochrome p-450 in male rats." *Journal of Toxicology and Environmental Health* vol. 71, no. 21, 2008: 1415–1429.

17. Shannon, M, et al. "In vitro bioassay investigations of the endocrine disrupting potential of steviol glycosides and their metabolite steviol, components of the natural sweetener Stevia." *Molecular Cell Endocrinology* vol. 427, 2016: 65–72.

18. Brickman, AM, et al. "Enhancing dentate gyrus function with dietary flavanols improves cognition in older adults." *Nature Neuroscience,* vol. 17, 2014: 1978–1803.

19. Wan, Ying, et al. "Effects of cocoa powder and dark chocolate on LDL oxidative susceptibility and prostaglandin concentrations in humans." *The American Journal of Clinical Nutrition,* vol. 74, no. 5, 2001: 596–602.

20. Gu, Y, and JD Lambert. "Modulation of metabolic syndrome-related inflammation by cocoa." *Molecular Nutrition and Food Research,* vol. 57, no. 6, 2013: 948–961.

21. Sies, H, et al. "Cocoa polyphenols and inflammatory mediators." *The American Journal of Clinical Nutrition* vol. 81 (1 Suppl), 2005: 304S–312S.

22. Hurst, WJ, et al. "Impact of fermentation, drying, roasting and Dutch processing on flavan-3-ol stereochemistry in cacao beans and cocoa ingredients." *Chemistry Central Journal* vol. 5, no. 53, 2011.

23. McCallum, L, et al. "The hidden hand of chloride in hypertension." *Pflugers Archives* vol. 467, no. 3, 2015: 595–603.

24. Popkin, BM, et al. "A new proposed guidance system for beverage consumption in the United States." *The American Journal of Clinical Nutrition* vol. 83, no. 3, 2006: 529–542.

— McCallum, L., et al. "Serum chloride is an independent predictor of mortality in hypertensive patients." *Hypertension* vol. 62, no. 5, 2013: 836–843.

25. Petrie, HJ, et al. "Caffeine ingestion increases the insulin response to an oral-glucose-tolerance test in obese men before and after weight loss." *The American Journal of Clinical Nutrition* vol. 80, no. 1, 2004: 22–28.

26. Tuomilehto, J, et al. "Coffee consumption and risk of type 2 diabetes mellitus among middle-aged Finnish men and women." *JAMA* vol. 291, no. 10, 2004: 1213–1219.

27. Nawrot, P, et al. "Effects of Caffeine on Human Health." *Food Additives and Contaminants,* vol. 20, no. 1, 2003: 1–30.

Chapter 5 Adopting the Paleo Feeding Pattern

1. United States Department of Agriculture, Food Safety and Inspection Service. "Water in meat and poultry." 6 Aug 2013. https://www.fsis.usda.gov/wps/portal/fsis/topics/food-safety-education/get-answers/food-safety-fact-sheets/meat-preparation/water-in-meat-and-poultry/ct_index%20

2. Center for Food Safety. "About Genetically Engineered Foods." Accessed 18 Jan 2017. http://www.centerforfoodsafety.org/issues/311/ge-foods/about-ge-foods

3. United States Food and Drug Administration. "Guidance for Industry: Voluntary Labeling Indicating Whether Foods Have or Have Not Been Derived from Genetically Engineered Plants." 1 July 2016. http://www.fda.gov/Food/GuidanceRegulation/GuidanceDocumentsRegulatoryInformation/LabelingNutrition/ucm059098.htm

4. Just Label It. "Labeling Around the World." Accessed 18 January 2017. http://www.justlabelit.org/right-to-know-center/labeling-around-the-world/

5. USDA National Organic Program. "Labeling Organic Products." *United States Department of Agriculture Agricultural Marketing Service,* Dec 2016. https://www.ams.usda.gov/sites/default/files/media/Labeling%20Organic%20Products.pdf

6. Worthington, V. "Nutritional quality of organic versus conventional fruits, vegetables, and grains." *The Journal of Alternative and Complementary Medicine* vol. 7, no. 2, 2001: 161–173.

7. American Heart Association. "Suggested Servings from Each Food Group." 11 January 2017. http://www.heart.org/HEARTORG/HealthyLiving/HealthyEating/Nutrition/Suggested-Servings-from-Each-Food-Group_UCM_318186_Article.jsp#.WHZbJrlSN-x

8. American Heart Association. "How Much Sodium Should I Eat Per Day?" Accessed 18 January 2017. https://sodiumbreakup.heart.org/how_much_sodium_should_i_eat?

9. Committee on Toxicity. "Phytoestrogens and Health." *Food Standards Agency,* May 2003. https://cot.food.gov.uk/sites/default/files/cot/phytoreport0503.pdf

10. Allen, LH. "Women's dietary calcium requirements are not increased by pregnancy or lactation." *The American Journal of Clinical Nutrition* vol. 67, no. 4, 1998: 591–592.

— Laskey, MA, et al. "Bone changes after three months of lactation: influence of calcium intake, breast-milk output, and vitamin D-receptor genotype." *The American Journal of Clinical Nutrition* vol. 67, no. 4, 1998: 685–692.

— Ritchie, LD, et al. "A longitudinal study of calcium homeostasis during human pregnancy and lactation and after resumption of menses." *The American Journal of Clinical Nutrition* vol. 67, no. 4, 1998: 693–701.

11. Holloway, M, and M Profet. "A Profile: Evolutionary Theories for Everyday Life." *Scientific American,* 1996.

Conclusion Healthy Lifespan and the Best of Both Worlds

1. Chernew, M, et al. "Understanding the improvement in disability free life expectancy in the U.S. elderly population." *National Bureau of Economic Research Working Paper,* no. 22306, June 2016.

2. Mokdad, AH, et al. "The spread of the obesity epidemic in the United States, 1991–1998." *JAMA,* vol. 282, no. 16, 1999: 1519–1522.

3. Fakhouri, THI, et al. "Prevalence of Obesity Among Older Adults in the United States, 2007–2010." *Centers for Disease Control and Prevention,* NCHS Data Brief, no. 106, 2012. https://www.cdc.gov/nchs/products/databriefs/db106.htm

4. Kochanek, KD, et al. "Deaths: Final Data for 2014." *National Vital Statistics Reports* vol. 65, no. 4, 2016. http://www.cdc.gov/nchs/data/nvsr/nvsr65/nvsr65_04.pdf.

5. Makary, MA, and M Daniel. "Medical error—the third leading cause of death in the US." *BMJ* vol. 353, 2016: i2139.

Appendix A Population Studies Supporting the Paleo Lifestyle

1. Department of Economic and Social Affairs. "2014 United Nations Demographic Yearbook." http://unstats.un.org/unsd/Demographic/products/dyb/dybsets/ 2014.pdf

2. United Nations ESCAP. Family Planning Programme, China Population Information and Research Centre (2002).

3. Helsing, E. "Traditional diets and disease patterns of the Mediterranean, circa 1960." *The American Journal of Clinical Nutrition* vol. 61, 6 Suppl, 1995: 1329S–1337S.

4. Kushi, LH. "Health implications of Mediterranean diets in light of contemporary knowledge. 1. Plant foods and dairy products." *The American Journal of Clinical Nutrition* vol. 61, 6 Suppl, 1995: 1407S–1415S.

5. WHO Health Statistics Annual. Geneva: World Health Organization, 1995.

6. Gjonça, A, and M Bobak. "Albanian paradox, another example of protective effect of Mediterranean lifestyle?" *Lancet* vol. 350, no. 9094, 1997: 1815–1817.

7. Office for National Statistics (UK).

8. World Health Organization (WHO) Report, June 5, 2000.

9. Phillipson, Connie. "Paleonutrition and modern nutrition." *World Review of Nutrition and Dietetics* vol. 81, 1997: 38–48.

10. Adams, Ruth. *Eating in Eden.* Emmaus, PA: Rodale Press, 1976.

11. Sinclair, HM. "Diet of Canadian Indians and Eskimos: Unusual Foods for Human Consumption." *Symposium* Proc 12, 1953: 69–82.

12. Rabinowitch, IM. "Clinical and other observations on Canadian Eskimos in the Eastern Arctic." *The Canadian Medical Association Journal,* vol. 34, no. 5, 1936: 487–501

13. Keenleyside, A. "Skeletal evidence of health and disease in pre-contact Alaskan Eskimos and Aleuts." *American Journal of Physical Anthropology* vol. 107, no. 1, 1998: 51–70.

— Sinclair, HM. "Diet of Canadian Indians and Eskimos: Unusual Foods for Human Consumption." *Symposium* Proc 12, 1953: 69–82.

14. Mann, GV, et al. "The health and nutritional status of Alaskan Eskimos." *The American Journal of Clinical Nutrition* vol. 11, no. 1, 1962: 31–76.

15. Mazess, RB, and W Mather. "Bone mineral content of North Alaskan Eskimos." *The American Journal of Clinical Nutrition* vol. 27, no. 9, 1974: 916–925.

16. Booyens, J, et al. "The Eskimo diet: Prophylactic effects ascribed to the balanced presence of natural cis unsaturated fatty acids and to the absence of unnatural trans and cis isomers of unsaturated fatty acids." *Medical Hypotheses* vol. 21, no. 4, 1986: 387–408.

17. Ho, KJ, et al. "Alaskan Arctic Eskimos: responses to a customary high fat diet." *The American Journal of Clinical Nutrition* vol. 25, no. 8, 1972: 737–745.

18. Bang, HO, et al. "Plasma lipid and lipoprotein pattern in Greenlandic west-coast Eskimos." *Lancet* vol. 297, no. 7710, 1971: 1143–1146.

19. Harman, D. "Free radical theory of aging: The 'free radical' diseases." *AGE* vol. 7, 1984: 111.

20. Bang, HO, et al. "Plasma lipid and lipoprotein pattern in Greenlandic west-coast Eskimos." *Lancet* vol. 297, no. 7710, 1971: 1143–1146.

21. Chern, Wen, et al. "Analysis of the food consumption of Japanese households." *Food and Agricultural Organization Economic and Social Development Paper* no. 152, 2003.

22. Grant, WB. "Trends in diet and Alzheimer's disease during the nutrition transition in Japan and developing countries." *Journal of Alzheimer's Disease* vol. 38, no. 3, 2014: 611–620.

23. Powles, J, et al. "Global, regional and national sodium intakes in 1990 and 2010: a systematic analysis of 24 h urinary sodium excretion and dietary surveys worldwide." *BMJ Open* vol. 3, no. 12, 2013: e003733.

— U.S. Department of Health and Human Services and U.S. Department of Agriculture. *Dietary Guidelines for Americans 2015–2020,* 8th ed, Dec. 2015. http://health.gov/dietaryguidelines/2015/guidelines/

24. Funatogawa, I, et al. "Trends in smoking and lung cancer mortality in Japan, by birth cohort, 1949–2010." *Bulletin of the World Health Organization* vol. 91, 2013: 332–340.

— Japan Tobacco Inc. "JT's annual survey finds 19.9% of Japanese adults are smokers." 30 July 2015. https://www.jt.com/media/news/2015/pdf/20150730_E01.pdf

25. Furst, B. "On the use of migration studies in the explanation of diseases of multifac-

torial causality: the risk of non-insulin-dependent diabetes in Japanese-Americans." *Nutrition Noteworthy* vol. 1, no. 1, 1998: Article 5.

— Marmot, MG and SL Syme. "Acculturation and coronary heart disease in Japanese-Americans." *American Journal of Epidemiology* vol. 104, no. 3, 1976: 225–247.

26. Kagawa, Y, et al. "Eicosapolyenoic acids of serum lipids of Japanese islanders with low incidence of cardiovascular diseases." *Journal of Nutritional Science and Vitaminology (Tokyo)* vol. 28, no. 4, 1982: 441–453.

27. Kagawa, Y, et al. "Eicosapolyenoic acids of serum lipids of Japanese islanders with low incidence of cardiovascular diseases." *Journal of Nutritional Science and Vitaminology (Tokyo)* vol. 28, no. 4, 1982: 441–453.

28. Cockerham, WC and Y Yamori. "Okinawa: an exception to the social gradient of life expectancy in Japan." *Asia Pacific Journal of Clinical Nutrition* vol. 10, no. 2, 2001: 154–158.

29. Xu, X, et al. "Tofu intake is associated with poor cognitive performance among community-dwelling elderly in China." *Journal of Alzheimer's Disease* vol. 43, no. 2, 2015: 669–675.

— Hogervorst, E, et al. "High tofu intake is associated with worse memory in elderly Indonesian men and women." *Dementia and Geriatric Cognitive Disorders* vol. 26, no. 1, 2008: 50–57.

— White, LR, et al. "Brain aging and midlife tofu consumption." *Journal of the American College of Nutrition* vol. 19, no. 2, 2000: 242–255.

30. Keys, A. "Coronary heart disease in seven countries." *Circulation* vol. 41, no. 4 Suppl, 1970: 1–211.

— Keys, A. *How to Eat Well and Stay Well the Mediterranean Way.* New York: Doubleday, 1975.

31. Renaud, S, et al. "Cretan Mediterranean diet for prevention of coronary heart disease." *The American Journal of Clinical Nutrition* vol. 61, no. 6 Suppl, 1995: 1360S–1367S.

About the Author

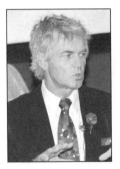

Geoff Bond graduated with honors in applied sciences from London University, and completed postgraduate professional qualifications in 1968. He spent his early career living and working in remote African villages, where he widened his earlier studies in anthropology, biochemistry, and evolutionary human development. Using both research and firsthand observation of tribal societies, by 1998, Bond had developed guidelines for living in harmony with the lifestyle that nature designed for us in Paleolithic times.

At the time he called it the Savanna Model, but subsequently it has become popularized under the term "Paleo." As such, Bond is one of the original pioneers of the Paleo precepts.

Bond is the author of *Deadly Harvest, Natural Eating,* and, with his wife Nicole, is the co-author of the cookbook *Paleo Harvest.* He also lectures extensively in both America and Europe, and is a frequent guest on television and radio shows.

Index